Chapter-(1)

Understanding Psoriasis:

1.1:What is Psoriasis?

1.2:Types of Psoriasis.

1.2:(a)Plaque Psoriasis.

1.2:(b)Guttate Psoriasis.

1.2:(c)Inverse Psoriasis.

1.2:(d)pustular Psoriasis.

1.2:(e)erythrodermic Psoriasis.

1.3)Causes and Triggers.

1.1:What is Psoriasis?

Psoriasis is a chronic autoimmune condition characterised by the rapid buildup of skin cel s, leading to the formation of thick, red, and scaly patches on the skin. This condition a ects approximately 2-3% of the global population, making it a prevalent dermatological disorder. While it primarily manifests on the skin, Patches of skin become scaly and in amed, most often on the scalp, elbows, or knees, but other parts of the body can be a ected as wel . psoriasis can also a ect nails, joints, and other parts of the body, signi cantly impacting an individual's physical and psychological wel -being.

Psoriasis is an autoimmune disease, which means that the immune system mistakenly attacks healthy tissue.

In the case of psoriasis, the immune system attacks the skin cel s, causing them to grow too quickly.This rapid growth leads to the buildup of skin cel s that we see as psoriasis plaques.

In addition to physical discomfort, psoriasis can have signi cant psychological and social impacts, leading to feelings of embarrassment, low self-esteem, and depression.Scientists do not ful y understand what causes psoriasis, but they know that it involves a mix of genetics and environmental factors.

While there is no cure for psoriasis, there are many e ective treatments available to manage the symptoms and improve quality of life.Having psoriasis carries the risk of getting other serious conditions, including:

• Psoriatic arthritis, a chronic form of arthritis that causes pain, swel ing, and sti ness of the joints and places where tendons and ligaments attach to bones (entheses).

• Cardiovascular events, such heart attacks and strokes.

• Mental health problems, such as low self-esteem, anxiety, and depression.

• People with psoriasis may also be more likely to get certain cancers, Crohn's disease, diabetes, metabolic syndrome, obesity, osteoporosis,

uveitis (in ammation of the middle of the eye), liver disease, and kidney disease.Anyone can get psoriasis, but it is more common in adults than in children. It a ects men and women equal y.

Symptoms of Psoriasis:

The symptoms of psoriasis can sometimes go through cycles, aring for a few weeks or months fol owed by periods when they subside or go into remission. There are many ways to treat psoriasis, and your treatment plan wil depend on the type and severity of disease.

Mild psoriasis can often be successful y treated with creams or ointments, while moderate and severe psoriasis may require pil s, injections, or light treatments. Managing common triggers, such as stress and skin injuries, can also help keep the symptoms under control.

Symptoms of psoriasis vary from person to person, but some common ones are:

• Patches of thick, red skin with silvery-white scales that itch or burn, typical y on the elbows, knees, scalp, trunk, palms, and soles of the feet.

• Dry, cracked skin that itches or bleeds.

• Thick, ridged, pitted nails.

• Poor sleep quality.

• Some patients have a related condition cal ed psoriatic arthritis, which can be characterised by sti , swol en, or painful joints; neck or back pain; or Achil es heel pain. If you have symptoms of psoriatic arthritis, it is important

to see your doctor soon because untreated psoriatic arthritis can lead to irreversible damage.

The symptoms of psoriasis can come and go. You may nd that there are times when your symptoms get worse, cal ed ares, fol owed by times when you feel better.

Causes of Psoriasis:

Psoriasis is an immune-mediated disease, which means that your body's immune system starts overacting and causing problems. If you have psoriasis, immune cel s become active and produce molecules that set o the rapid production of skin cel s. This is why skin in people with the disease is in amed and scaly. Scientists do not ful y understand what triggers the faulty immune cel activation, but they know that it involves a combination of genetics and environmental factors.

Many people with psoriasis have a family history of the disease, and researchers have pinpointed some of the genes that may contribute to its development. Many of them play a role in the function of the immune system.

Some external factors that may increase the chances of developing psoriasis include:

• Infections, especial y streptococcal and HIV

infections.

• Certain medicines, such as drugs for treating heart disease, malaria, or mental health problems.

• Smoking.

• Obesity.

1.2):Di erent Types Of Psoriasis: There are a few types of psoriasis. While some are similar, they can also have di erent symptoms and treatments. Each type a ects a di erent area of your body.Each type of psoriasis has di erent signs and symptoms and can look di erent on each person. It's possible to have more than one type at a time. Psoriasis occurs when the life cycle of skin cel s speeds up, resulting in a rapid buildup of rough, dead skin cel s.

These skin cel s build up and form dry, scaly patches.

Knowing which kind of psoriasis you have helps you and your doctor make a treatment plan. Most people have only one type at a time. Sometimes, after your symptoms go away, a new form of psoriasis may crop up.

2.1:(a)Plaque Psoriasis:

Plaque psoriasis, also known as psoriasis vulgaris, is the most common form of psoriasis, accounting for approximately 80% of cases. It is a chronic autoimmune condition characterised by the rapid growth and shedding of skin cel s, resulting in the formation of raised, red patches covered with a silvery-white scale. This condition can signi cantly impact an individual's quality of life due to its physical discomfort, emotional distress, and potential complications.

Pathophysiology:

The pathophysiology of plaque psoriasis involves a complex interplay of genetic, environmental, and immunological factors. Genetic predisposition plays a signi cant role, with certain gene variants, such as those related to the immune system and skin barrier function, increasing the risk of developing the condition. Environmental triggers, such as stress, infections, injury to the skin, and certain medications, can exacerbate or precipitate are-ups in susceptible individuals.

Central to the development of plaque psoriasis is dysregulation of the immune system, particularly the involvement of T lymphocytes and in ammatory cytokines. In ammation is triggered by the release of pro-in ammatory molecules, leading to hyperproliferation of keratinocytes in the epidermis and abnormal di erentiation of skin cel s. This results in the characteristic features of psoriatic plaques, including erythema, scaling, and thickening of the skin.

Clinical Presentation:

Plaque psoriasis typical y presents as wel -de ned, erythematous plaques covered with silvery-white scales.

These plaques can vary in size and shape, ranging from smal patches to large, con uent areas. They commonly appear on extensor surfaces such as the elbows, knees, scalp, and lower back but can a ect any part of the body, including the nails and mucous membranes. The lesions may be asymptomatic or associated with

itching, burning, or pain, depending on their location and severity.

Psoriasis is a skin disease that affects about 8

million Americans. It comes in several forms.

Plaque psoriasis is the most common.

Plaques are raised red patches covered with a whitish buildup of dead skins cel s cal ed scale. They usual y show up on your elbows, knees, scalp, and lower back, but you can have them anywhere. Plaques often itch or hurt.

Causes of plaque psoriasis:

Doctors aren't sure why people get plaque psoriasis. It's considered an autoimmune disease. That means your immune system attacks healthy cel s as if it's ghting an infection. This causes new skin cel s to grow much faster than normal, and they build up in thick patches.

Whether you get plaque psoriasis depends on your genes and your health history:

Plaque psoriasis is the most common form of psoriasis.

It commonly appears as red, silvery-scaly plaques, as shown here on this male's hands. A chronic disease, it goes through cycles of ares and remissions.

- **Heredity**.

Psoriasis seems to run in families. About one out of three people with psoriasis report having a relative with psoriasis. About 10% of people are born with genes that make them likely to get psoriasis. But only about 3% of people get

the disease. Stil , If both parents have psoriasis, a child has about a 50% chance of getting the disease.

- **Triggers**. Something has to happen to start your immune system's reaction. Sometimes, it's an injury to your skin or a bad sunburn. It could be a certain medicine, like lithium or malaria drugs. An infection, particularly strep, can bring on psoriasis. So can high levels of stress, smoking, or drinking alcohol.

Psoriasis isn't contagious. It can't be spread by touch or other close contact.

People with psoriasis tend to have other conditions that cause in ammation, like Crohn's disease, diabetes, metabolic syndrome, fatty liver disease, and obesity. If you have it, you may be more likely to get heart disease, depression, and a kind of eye disease cal ed uveitis. You also have as much as a 1-in-3 chance of getting psoriatic arthritis, which causes joint pain, sti ness, and swel ing, and joint deformity.

Diagnosis of Plaque Psoriasis:

The diagnosis of plaque psoriasis is primarily based on clinical evaluation, including a thorough medical history and physical examination. Characteristic features such as the presence of plaques with silvery scales and a symmetrical distribution aid in distinguishing psoriasis from other skin conditions. In

some cases, a skin biopsy may be performed to con rm the diagnosis and rule out other disorders.

A dermatologist (skin doctor) can usual y tel if you have plaque psoriasis just by talking with you about your medical history and looking at your skin. But since psoriasis can look like eczema and other skin diseases, diagnosing it can be di cult. In some cases, your doctor may need to do a biopsy. They'l take a tiny sample of your skin and look at the cel s under a microscope.

Types of Plaque Psoriasis;

There are a number of terms that help doctors to di erentiate one type of plaque psoriasis from another: **Small-plaque psoriasis:** This version causes lots of little lesions, each one no bigger than a few centimetres.

They may remain separate or they could merge. The crusty parts on top are pink with a ner grain and thinner crust than in large plaque psoriasis. A family history of psoriasis is less common in this version of the condition.

Smal -plaque psoriasis can happen at any age, but it's more common after age 40. It often responds wel to phototherapy.

Large-plaque psoriasis: Here, the lesions are thicker and often larger with edges that are more clear than in smal -plaque psoriasis. The crusty parts are red rather than pink and show a whitish-silvery scale.

Large-plaque psoriasis can emerge anytime but is more common in those younger than 40. Some studies link the condition to metabolic syndrome. (Metabolic syndrome is when you have some combination of obesity, high cholesterol, high blood sugar, or high blood pressure.) It's harder to treat than smal -plaque psoriasis, and it's more likely to run in families.

Unstable plaque psoriasis:

In unstable psoriasis, the plaques of psoriasis lose their sharp, clear edges as they enlarge and sometimes join together. New plaques may appear too.

Chronic, stable plaque psoriasis: This is the most common form of plaque psoriasis and psoriasis in general. Lesions tend to stick around or reemerge after the rst outbreak. The most common areas are the elbows, knees, torso, and head and scalp, though there may be other areas too.

Plaques tend to emerge on both sides of your body. For example, if they show up on one elbow, they wil appear on the other one as wel .

Treatment of Plaque Psoriasis:

The management of plaque psoriasis aims to al eviate symptoms, reduce in ammation, and prevent are-ups while improving the patient's quality of life. Treatment approaches may vary depending on the severity of the

condition, individual patient factors, and treatment preferences. Common treatment modalities include: **a)Topical Medications**:

If you have only a few plaques, your doctor wil probably try a prescription cream rst. You put these directly on your skin. They help with in ammation or slow the growth of skin cel s. Examples include anthralin, ro umilast (Zoryve), corticosteroids, (Vtama), vitamin A, and vitamin D. You can also try over-the-counter topical medicines. Salicylic acid and coal tar are approved to treat psoriasis. Other ingredients may soothe itch and remove scale, including aloe vera, capsaicin, jojoba, and zinc pyrithione. Topical emol ients that you put on after a shower or bath can help keep your skin moist.

Corticosteroids, vitamin D analogs, retinoids, and calcineurin inhibitors are often used topical y to reduce in ammation and promote skin normalisation.

What to Expect With Topical Treatment for Plaque Psoriasis:

Psoriasis is a lifelong condition that comes and goes in ares, and the key to managing it is the right treatment.

Your dermatologist wil help you nd a therapy based on:

- How bad your symptoms are

- Which part of your body psoriasis a ects

- Which form of the condition you have

Did You Know?

Topicals work in two ways: They ease in ammation and slow the overactive skin cel growth that causes psoriasis. Topicals are a common type of psoriasis medicine that you apply to your skin to soothe irritation and scaling.

If you have mild psoriasis, your doctor may suggest an over the counter treatment such as:

- *Moisturisers*

- *Creams or ointments with hydrocortisone*

- *Coal tar products*

- *Scale softeners with salicylic acid*

Treatments for serious symptoms are more targeted.

They include prescription topical medicines that come in the form of a cream, ointment, or shampoo. You may use them in combination with other types of treatment. Here's a closer look at what you can expect with topicals.

i)How Should You Apply a Topical?

You'l apply a topical to the psoriasis-a ected area once or twice a day. With some products, it's essential to test a smal area of skin (cal ed a patch test) to make sure the medication won't cause further irritation.

If you're using a topical steroid, apply only a smal amount to the areas of your skin impacted by psoriasis.

The standard amount is one ngertip to cover the area of about two adult-sized palms. Unless your doctor says it's OK, don't apply a topical steroid near your eye area. This can cause eye problems such as cataracts and glaucoma.

ii)What Are the Side E ects of Topicals?

Side e ects of topicals can range from mild to serious.

They vary depending on the type of medication you use. Possible negative reactions include: **Topical steroids**

- Thinning of skin

- Skin colour changes

- Bruising without much e ort

- Stretch marks

10

- Enlarged blood vessels

If you apply a topical steroid to a broad area or use it for an extended amount of time, there's also a chance it wil absorb through your skin and a ect your internal organs.

Non-steroid topicals

- Irritated skin

- A stinging or burning feeling

- Dry, itchy, peeling skin

- Rash

- Worsened psoriasis

- Sun sensitivity and a higher chance of skin tumours

- Too much calcium in your pee

- Raised bumps around your hair

- Nose and throat pain or swel ing fol icles

- Headache

- Diarrhoea

- Trouble fal ing or staying asleep (insomnia)

- Feeling sick to your stomach (nausea)

- Upper respiratory tract infection

- Urinary tract infection (UTI)

iii)Over the counter topicals

Many over-the-counter psoriasis products contain the ingredient salicylic acid. It works by softening, lifting, and removing psoriasis scales. If you leave it on your skin for too long, though, it can irritate the skin. And if you use it on a large area of skin, your body may soak up too much of it, which can cause further health problems.

Another over-the-counter product, coal tar, also comes with possible side effects such as skin irritation, dryness, and colour changes. You could also become more sensitive to sunlight, so wear sunscreen and protective clothing and stay out of the sun as much as possible while using this product.

iv)Combining Topicals or a Topical With Another Type of Treatment:

Serious psoriasis symptoms may require a combination of treatments. Your dermatologist could suggest applying a topical while also using phototherapy (light therapy) or taking an immunosuppressant, biologic, or smal molecule inhibitor.

You may also nd that some topical formulations work better on certain areas of your body. For example, people often use foam medication for scalp psoriasis and a lotion on their bodies.

Even when you nd the right combination, it's stil likely that your psoriasis wil return. But you'l now have a treatment that works wel when your symptoms come back.

v)How Long Will You Use a Topical?

Topical steroids range in strength from strong (most potent) to weak (least potent). How long you'l use these medications depends on their strength. You should use super high-potency topical steroids for no more than 3 straight weeks and high- to medium-strength for 12 weeks.

If you need treatment for a longer period, talk to your doctor. They may suggest that you use a high-strength topical steroid less frequently or have you switch to a milder treatment. Once your symptoms have cleared up, you can stop using the medication.

There are other types of topicals, like those without steroids, and ones you can buy over the counter. Talk to your doctor about how long you should use these treatments, and careful y fol ow al instructions included with the medication

vi)When Should You Stop Taking a Topical?

Finding the right treatment, or combination of treatments, can be a time-consuming process. Sticking with treatment can be hard, but not fol owing through is one of the biggest barriers to success. It's crucial to fol ow your doctor's instructions to see improvement in your symptoms.

It's also important to keep using a topical steroid until you get your doctor's OK to taper o the medication.

If you suddenly stop, it can cause your psoriasis to get worse. It can also trigger a side e ect known as topical steroid withdrawal (TSW). TSW happens when you abruptly stop taking a topical steroid instead of tapering o . It can cause a burning feeling, aking, swel ing, and other skin symptoms

b)Phototherapy or light therapy: Ultraviolet (UV) light therapy, including narrowband UVB and psoralen plus UVA (PUVA) therapy, can

help reduce in ammation and slow down the rapid growth of skin cel s.

If the rash is more widespread, your doctor may treat it with ultraviolet light. This is done at their o ce or with a special box you can keep at home. You may also get relief by going out in the sun, but this can raise your risk of skin cancer. Watch how long you spend outside, and cover up or put sunscreen on places where you don't have plaques.

c)Systemic medications: For more severe cases, systemic medications such as methotrexate, cyclosporine, acitretin, and biologic agents (e.g., TNF-alpha inhibitors, IL-17 inhibitors) may be prescribed to target the underlying immune dysfunction.

If you have a severe case of plaque psoriasis, you may need medicines that work throughout your body. They calm your immune system or make your skin cel s grow more slowly. But they can cause serious side e ects, like depression, aggressive thoughts, liver problems, or a higher risk of skin cancer. You take systemic drugs like acitretin, cyclosporine, and methotrexate by pil , or your doctor wil give you a shot.Another kind of systemic drug also targets your immune system.

Biologic drugs used to treat psoriasis include:

• Adalimumab (Humira)

• Brodalumab (Siliq)

• Certolizumab-pegol (Cimzia)

• Deucravacitinib (Soty Ktu)

• Etanercept (Enbrel)

• Golimumab (Simponi) and Abatacept (Orencia) (for psoriatic arthritis)

• Guselkumab (Tremfya)

• In iximab (Avsola, In ectra, Remicade)

• Ixekizumab (Taltz Autoinjector, Taltz Syringe).

They're given in a shot, pil , or through a vein in your arm. They a ect a speci c type of immune cel or keep certain proteins from causing in ammation. But these drugs can make it harder for you to ght an infection.

d)Lifestyle modi cations:

Avoiding triggers such as stress, smoking, excessive alcohol consumption, and certain medications can help reduce the frequency and severity of are-ups.

Additional y, maintaining a healthy lifestyle with regular exercise, balanced nutrition, and adequate hydration can support overal skin health.

Psoriasis can't be cured. You'l probably go through cycles where the rash looks better and then ares up again. The goal of treatment is fewer and less severe are-ups.

You may get medicine to put on your skin, you may take pil s, or your doctor may recommend a combination of those. Treatment options include:

What You Can Do: Most people who get plaque psoriasis have it for the rest of their lives. You can do a few things to deal with it better:

Avoid triggers. Things like stress and smoking don't cause psoriasis. But they can make it worse. Try to gure out what triggers your are-ups. You may be a ected by:

- Alcohol

- Al ergies

- Cold, dry weather

- Hormones.

Watch your diet. There's no proof that speci c foods make a di erence with psoriasis. But losing weight may keep your symptoms at bay, so it makes sense to eat healthy. And a diet low in fatty meat and dairy products and high in sh and colourful fruits and vegetables may help with in ammation.

Take care of your skin:

A good moisturiser can keep plaques soft and make you less itchy. Avoid harsh soaps. A bath with col oidal oatmeal or Epsom salts can also soothe your skin. Try using medicated shampoo for scales on your scalp. A cream with strontium can also help relieve itching.

Get support:

Plaque psoriasis can take an emotional tol . You may feel self-conscious about the way it looks or overwhelmed by what it takes to manage it. Many people with psoriasis become depressed. If you think you need some help, talk with your doctor about therapy or medication. It also helps to talk with people who understand what you're going through and can o er ways to cope.

Complications:

Plaque psoriasis is associated with various complications, both physical and psychological.

Physical complications:

may include psoriatic arthritis, which a ects up to 30%

of patients with psoriasis and can lead to joint damage and disability if left untreated. Other complications may include secondary bacterial or fungal infections, metabolic syndrome, cardiovascular disease, and an increased risk of certain malignancies.

Psychosocial Impact:

Beyond its physical manifestations, plaque psoriasis can have a profound impact on patients' mental health and quality of life. The visible nature of the lesions may lead to feelings of embarrassment, self-consciousness, and social isolation, contributing to anxiety, depression, and decreased self-esteem. Managing the psychosocial aspects of psoriasis is an essential component of comprehensive care, often requiring psychological support, counsel ing, and education.

Conclusion:

Plaque psoriasis is a chronic autoimmune condition characterised by the development of raised, red plaques covered with silvery scales. Its pathophysiology involves immune dysregulation, genetic predisposition, and environmental triggers. Diagnosis is primarily clinical, and treatment aims to al eviate symptoms, reduce in ammation, and prevent complications. Despite advances in therapy, plaque psoriasis remains a chal enging condition to manage, highlighting the importance of a multidisciplinary approach to care that addresses both the physical and psychosocial aspects of the disease.

1.2:(b)Guttate Psoriasis:

Guttate psoriasis is a type of psoriasis that shows up on your skin as red, scaly, smal , teardrop-shaped spots. It doesn't normal y leave a scar. You usual y get it as a child or young adult. Less than a third of people with psoriasis have this type. It's not as common as plaque psoriasis. This variant comprises approximately 8% of al psoriasis cases and often presents in childhood or early adulthood.

It's an autoimmune disease, meaning your body treats your own cel s like invaders and attacks them. You

might get it only once, or you could have several are-ups. In some cases, this type of psoriasis doesn't go away. With the help of your doctor, you can nd a treatment to keep your symptoms under control.

Symptoms of Guttate

Psoriasis:

The spots you get from guttate psoriasis aren't as thick as the ones from plaque psoriasis. You can sometimes have both kinds of psoriasis at once. You probably would get them on your arms, legs, and upper body.

It can sometimes spread from there to your face, ears, and scalp. But it doesn't show up on your palms, the soles of your feet, or nails like other forms of psoriasis can. You're more likely to have a are-up during the winter, when the air is dry. Your symptoms may clear up more quickly in summer.

Stages of Guttate Psoriasis:

There are three:

Mild. Only a few spots cover about 3% of your skin.

Moderate. Lesions cover about 3%-10% of your skin.

Severe. Lesions cover 10% or more of your body and could cover your entire body.

The stage can also be based on how much they interfere with your daily life and activities. For example, psoriasis on your face or scalp can a ect only 2%-3% of your total body surface area, but it could be classi ed as severe because it a ects your appearance and livelihood.

Psoriasis on your hands might only cover 2% total body

surface area, but could a ect your livelihood if you work with your hands. In that case it would be classi ed as moderate to severe.

Causes and Triggers of Guttate Psoriasis: An outbreak is usual y triggered by a bacterial infection

-- typical y streptococcus (strep throat). It sets o an immune system reaction that causes the spots on your skin.

In some cases, guttate psoriasis is genetic. If someone in your family has it, your chances of getting it go up.

Other triggers include:

- Upper respiratory infections

- Sinus infections

- Flu

- Tonsil itis

- Stress

- Cuts, burns, or bites on your skin

- Some drugs you take (antimalarials and beta-blockers)

Understanding the pathophysiology, clinical features, diagnosis, treatment, and potential complications of guttate psoriasis is crucial for e ective management of this skin condition.

Pathophysiology:

Guttate psoriasis shares common immunologic pathways with other forms of psoriasis, involving genetic predisposition, environmental triggers, and immune system dysregulation. Genetic factors

contribute signi cantly, with speci c gene variants linked to psoriasis susceptibility. Environmental triggers, such as streptococcal infections (particularly streptococcal throat infections), stress, and skin injuries, can provoke an immune response that leads to the development of guttate psoriasis in genetical y predisposed individuals.

The condition is characterised by an accelerated turnover of skin cel s, leading to the rapid proliferation and shedding of cel s in the epidermis. In ammatory cytokines, particularly tumour necrosis factor-alpha (TNF-alpha) and interleukins, play a central role in the development of guttate psoriasis lesions.

Clinical Presentation:

Guttate psoriasis is distinguished by the appearance of numerous smal , red, and scaly lesions resembling water droplets. These lesions are typical y 1 to 10

mil imetres in diameter and may cover large areas of the body, including the trunk, limbs, and sometimes the face and scalp. The individual lesions are often separate but may coalesce to form larger plaques.

Unlike other forms of psoriasis, guttate psoriasis is commonly triggered by streptococcal infections, and the onset of lesions may fol ow an upper respiratory infection or streptococcal pharyngitis. The condition may manifest suddenly and resolve on its own, but in some cases, it can evolve into chronic plaque psoriasis.

Diagnosis of Guttate Psoriasis: Your doctor wil want to know your medical history, especial y what kinds of medications you may be taking. They'l look at your skin. Usual y, a physical exam gives your doctor enough information to diagnose or rule out guttate psoriasis.

Diagnosing guttate psoriasis involves a thorough clinical examination, medical history review, and consideration of potential triggers. The distinctive appearance of smal , drop-shaped lesions is a key diagnostic feature. Additional y, a throat swab or blood test may be conducted to identify streptococcal infections, aiding in the con rmation of a potential triggering factor.

Skin biopsy is rarely necessary but may be performed in atypical cases or when the diagnosis is uncertain.

Histopathological examination typical y reveals characteristic features of psoriasis, such as hyperkeratosis, parakeratosis, and an in ammatory in ltrate in the dermis.

Treatment for Guttate Psoriasis: In most cases, an outbreak of guttate psoriasis lasts 2 to 3 weeks. But your doctor may want to treat your symptoms and help prevent other infections in your body.

The management of guttate psoriasis includes addressing both the acute are-ups and potential underlying triggers. Treatment strategies may include: **Topical therapies or Medical treatments:**

There are several over-the-counter or prescription options for the itchy, aky skin, as wel as the dryness and swel ing. They include:

- Cortisone cream for itching and swel ing

- Dandru shampoo for your scalp

- Lotions with coal tar to soothe your skin

- Moisturisers

- Prescription medicines with vitamin A

- If your case is more serious, your doctor may give you a prescription to take by mouth.

These include:

- Corticosteroids

- Biologics (guselkumab, ixekizumab)

- Apremilast (Otezla)

- Deucravacitib (Soty Ktu)

- Methotrexate

- Corticosteroids and vitamin D analogs are commonly used to reduce in ammation and scale. Emol ients can help soothe and hydrate the skin.

Phototherapy:

Also known as light therapy, this is another option.

Your doctor wil shine ultraviolet light onto your skin during this treatment. They may also give you medication to make your skin react more quickly to light. Sometimes, just going out into the sunshine can help.Ultraviolet B (UVB) phototherapy, especial y narrowband UVB, can be e ective in control ing guttate psoriasis. Exposure to natural sunlight may also

have bene cial e ects but it should be done on doctor's advice.

Antibiotics:

In cases triggered by streptococcal infections, antibiotics may be prescribed to eliminate the bacterial infection and potential y improve psoriasis symptoms.

Why Antibiotics?

Guttate is a type of psoriasis. It's the most common type after plaque psoriasis. It often starts in children or young adults and usual y appears as smal , red, teardrop-shaped spots on your arms, legs, and torso.

Systemic medications: In severe or persistent cases, oral medications such as methotrexate or cyclosporine may be considered. Biologic agents targeting speci c immune pathways can also be used in select cases.

Prognosis and Complications:

Guttate psoriasis often has a better prognosis than other forms of psoriasis, and many cases resolve spontaneously. However, individuals with guttate psoriasis may be at an increased risk of developing chronic plaque psoriasis later in life. Complications can include psychological distress due to the visible nature of the lesions and potential long-term skin changes.

Conclusion:

Guttate psoriasis is a distinctive variant characterised by smal , drop-shaped lesions that often fol ow streptococcal infections. Its pathophysiology involves genetic predisposition, immune system dysregulation, and environmental triggers. Diagnosis is primarily

clinical, with treatment options ranging from topical therapies to systemic medications. Prognosis is general y favourable, but careful management is essential to address acute episodes, potential complications, and the overal wel -being of individuals with guttate psoriasis.

1.2(c)Inverse Psoriasis:

Inverse psoriasis, also known as intertriginous or exural psoriasis, is a type of psoriasis that manifests in the folds of the skin. Unlike the more common plaque psoriasis characterised by raised, scaly patches, inverse psoriasis appears as smooth, red lesions in areas where skin surfaces touch or rub together. These regions commonly include the armpits, groyne, buttocks, and beneath the breasts.

Inverse psoriasis is prone to moisture and friction, making it distinct from other forms of psoriasis. Due to its location, it can be more chal enging to diagnose and may be mistaken for other skin conditions like fungal infections. Symptoms often include red, in amed skin with a shiny and smooth appearance. It may be associated with discomfort, itching, and a burning sensation.

Treatment for inverse psoriasis typical y involves topical corticosteroids, calcineurin inhibitors, and antifungal medications to address secondary infections.

Maintaining good hygiene, keeping the a ected areas dry, and avoiding irritants can help manage symptoms.

In some cases, systemic medications or phototherapy may be considered for more severe or widespread cases.

As with other types of psoriasis, it's essential for individuals with inverse psoriasis to work closely with healthcare professionals to develop an appropriate treatment plan tailored to their speci c needs.

Inverse psoriasis, also known as intertriginous or exural psoriasis, is a variant of psoriasis characterised by smooth, red lesions that develop in skin folds and creases. Unlike the more common plaque psoriasis, which presents as raised, scaly patches on the extensor surfaces of the body, inverse psoriasis a ects areas where skin surfaces touch or rub together, such as the armpits, groyne, buttocks, and beneath the breasts.

This type of psoriasis is often overlooked or misdiagnosed due to its location and appearance, leading to delays in treatment and management.

Clinical Presentation:

Inverse psoriasis lesions appear as bright red patches of skin that lack the typical scaling seen in other forms of psoriasis. The a ected areas may have a smooth, shiny appearance due to the moisture and friction present in skin folds. Patients commonly experience discomfort, itching, and a burning sensation, particularly in areas prone to sweating. Since these symptoms overlap with those of fungal infections and other dermatoses, accurate diagnosis can be chal enging and may require a comprehensive evaluation by a dermatologist.

Trigger Factors: The exact cause of psoriasis, including its inverse form, remains unclear. However, various factors are believed to contribute to its development and exacerbation.

Genetic predisposition, immune dysregulation, environmental triggers, and alterations in skin microbiota are among the factors implicated in the pathogenesis of psoriasis. Inverse psoriasis, in particular, may be exacerbated by friction, sweating, heat, and microbial infections in skin folds. Obesity and other comorbid conditions, such as metabolic syndrome and autoimmune diseases, can also in uence disease severity and treatment outcomes.

Diagnosis:

Diagnosing inverse psoriasis requires a thorough clinical examination, including a detailed medical history and physical assessment of the a ected areas.

Dermatologists may perform a skin biopsy to con rm the diagnosis and rule out other conditions that mimic inverse psoriasis, such as candidiasis or seborrheic dermatitis. In some cases, additional diagnostic tests, such as fungal cultures or imaging studies, may be necessary to di erentiate between psoriasis and other dermatoses.

Management Strategies:

Topical Therapies:

The primary goal of treating inverse psoriasis is to al eviate symptoms, reduce in ammation, and prevent secondary infections. Topical corticosteroids,

calcineurin inhibitors, and vitamin D analogs are commonly used as rst-line therapies for mild to moderate cases of inverse psoriasis. These medications help suppress immune-mediated in ammation and restore the integrity of the skin barrier. Patients should apply topical treatments sparingly to avoid skin atrophy and monitor for adverse e ects, such as tachyphylaxis and al ergic reactions.

Moisturisers and Barrier Creams: Emol ients and barrier creams play a crucial role in managing inverse psoriasis by hydrating the skin and minimising friction-induced irritation. Patients should use fragrance-free moisturisers and non-comedogenic emol ients regularly to maintain skin hydration and integrity. Barrier creams containing zinc oxide or petroleum jel y can create a protective layer over a ected areas, reducing moisture loss and preventing skin breakdown. Proper skin care practices, including gentle cleansing and pat-drying, are essential for preventing exacerbations and promoting healing in inverse psoriasis.

Systemic Therapies:

In cases of severe or refractory inverse psoriasis, systemic therapies may be warranted to achieve disease control and improve quality of life. Oral medications, such as methotrexate, cyclosporine, and acitretin, target key in ammatory pathways involved in psoriasis pathogenesis. Biologic agents, including tumour necrosis factor-alpha (TNF-alpha) inhibitors,

interleukin (IL)-17 inhibitors, and IL-23 inhibitors, o er targeted therapy by blocking speci c cytokines implicated in psoriasis progression. These systemic agents are reserved for patients with moderate to severe inverse psoriasis who have failed conventional treatments or are unable to tolerate them due to adverse e ects.

Phototherapy:

Phototherapy, or light therapy, is another treatment option for patients with inverse psoriasis who do not respond to topical or systemic therapies. Narrowband ultraviolet B (UVB) phototherapy and psoralen plus ultraviolet A (PUVA) therapy have demonstrated e cacy in reducing in ammation and inducing remission in psoriatic lesions. Phototherapy works by modulating immune responses and promoting apoptosis of activated T cel s in the skin. Regular monitoring and dose adjustments are necessary to minimise the risk of phototoxicity and long-term adverse e ects associated with prolonged UV exposure.

Lifestyle Modi cations and Patient Education: Weight Management:

Maintaining a healthy weight through diet and exercise is essential for managing inverse psoriasis, as obesity can exacerbate in ammation and worsen disease severity.

Patients with psoriasis should adopt a balanced diet rich in fruits, vegetables, whole grains, and lean proteins while limiting intake of processed foods, sugary beverages, and high-fat meals. Regular physical

activity, such as walking, swimming, or yoga, can help reduce systemic in ammation, improve cardiovascular health, and enhance overal wel -being in patients with psoriasis.

Stress Reduction:

Psychological stress has been implicated as a trigger for psoriasis ares and exacerbations. Stress management techniques, such as mindfulness meditation, deep breathing exercises, and cognitive-behavioural therapy, can help patients cope with the emotional burden of living with a chronic skin condition. Encouraging social support networks and engaging in enjoyable activities can also promote resilience and reduce the impact of stress on psoriasis management.

Skincare Practices:

Educating patients about proper skin care practices is essential for preventing complications and optimising treatment outcomes in inverse psoriasis. Patients should be advised to avoid harsh soaps, abrasive scrubs, and perfumed products that can irritate sensitive skin and exacerbate in ammation. Instead, they should opt for gentle cleansers, hypoal ergenic moisturisers, and fragrance-free cosmetics formulated for sensitive skin.

Regular monitoring by a dermatologist and adherence to prescribed treatment regimens are crucial for achieving long-term remission and improving quality of life in patients with inverse psoriasis.

Conclusion:

Inverse psoriasis presents unique chal enges in diagnosis and management due to its distinct clinical features and predilection for intertriginous areas. A multidisciplinary approach involving dermatologists, primary care physicians, and al ied healthcare professionals is essential for providing comprehensive care and addressing the complex needs of patients with inverse psoriasis. By implementing evidence-based treatment strategies, promoting healthy lifestyle modi cations, and fostering patient education and support, healthcare providers can empower individuals with inverse psoriasis to achieve optimal outcomes and regain control of their skin health and overal wel -being.

1.2:(d)Pustular Psoriasis:

Pustular psoriasis is a skin disease. You'l see white bumps l ed with pus near or inside red skin blotches.

These are cal ed pustules. They can hurt and be scaly, aky, or itchy.

It's most likely to a ect:

- The palms of your hands

- The soles of your feet

- Your ngers and toes

Even though you see pus in your bumps, it's not an infection. You can't catch pustular psoriasis from someone else or give it to others.

Pustular psoriasis usual y happens to adults. It's rare for kids to have it. But it can run in families.

You can get pustular psoriasis on its own or with another kind of psoriasis cal ed plaque psoriasis.

Types and Symptoms of pustular psoriasis: There are multiple types of pustular psoriasis. They're based on where the blister outbreaks are or how fast they popped up.

Palmoplantar pustulosis (PPP): Blisters form on smal areas of your body, usual y your palms or the soles of your feet. These pus-l ed spots can turn brown, peel o , or crust over. Your skin can crack, too.

This type of psoriasis may come and go. People who smoke are more likely to get this form.

Acropustulosis:

Smal , very painful lesions pop up on your ngertips or toes. The pain can make it hard to use your ngers or toes. In rare cases, it can cause nail or even bone damage.

Generalised or Von Zumbusch: Red, painful, tender skin blotches show up over a wide area of your body, and pus- l ed blisters pop up soon after. Your skin may be very itchy. You also might be very tired or have a fever, chil s, dehydration, nausea, weak muscles, headache, joint pain, a fast pulse, or

weight loss. This is a rare, serious disease. See your doctor right away if you have these symptoms.

Causes and Triggers:

Psoriasis is an autoimmune disease. Your immune system usual y sends white blood cel s to ght disease in your body. But in this case, they attack your healthy skin by mistake.

A few things can trigger psoriasis ares:

● Medications, such as steroids

● Something that irritates your skin, like a topical cream or harsh skin care product

● Too much sunlight

● Stress

● Pregnancy

- Infection

- Hormones

- A mutation, or change, in one of two speci c genes (IL36RN or CARD14) may make you more likely to get pustular psoriasis. If you have one of these gene mutations, one of those triggers could set o a are.

The exact cause of pustular psoriasis remains elusive, but it is believed to involve a complex interplay of genetic predisposition, immune dysfunction, and environmental triggers. Genetic factors play a signi cant role, as individuals with a family history of psoriasis are at a higher risk of developing the condition. Dysregulation of the immune system,

particularly involving T cel s and cytokines, contributes to the in ammatory cascade observed in psoriasis.

Environmental triggers such as stress, infections, medications, and certain lifestyle factors can exacerbate symptoms or trigger are-ups in susceptible individuals.

Diagnosis:

You'l see a dermatologist (a skin doctor) who wil ask about your symptoms, your medical history, and any family history of psoriasis.

They may need to take a smal sample of your in amed skin to look at under a microscope. That's cal ed a biopsy.

If you have a severe are, they may also test your blood for signs of high white blood cel counts; signs that your kidney and liver are working the way they should; and whether you have healthy levels of electrolytes, calcium, and phosphate.

Diagnosing pustular psoriasis requires a thorough evaluation by a dermatologist or healthcare professional. Clinical examination of the skin lesions, along with a review of the patient's medical history, helps in establishing a preliminary diagnosis. In some cases, additional tests may be recommended to rule out other skin conditions or assess the severity of systemic involvement. These tests may include skin biopsies,

blood tests to evaluate in ammatory markers, and imaging studies to monitor for complications such as joint in ammation (psoriatic arthritis) or organ involvement.

Clinical Presentation:

Pustular psoriasis is characterised by the presence of pus- l ed blisters, known as pustules, on the skin.

These pustules typical y appear on red, in amed skin and can be localised to speci c areas or spread across large portions of the body. The condition can manifest in di erent forms, including generalised pustular psoriasis (GPP), palmoplantar pustulosis (PPP), and acrodermatitis continua of Hal opeau (ACH). GPP is the most severe form, presenting with widespread pustules accompanied by systemic symptoms such as fever, chil s, and malaise.

Treatment:

The management of pustular psoriasis aims to al eviate symptoms, reduce in ammation, and prevent complications. Treatment strategies may vary depending on the subtype and severity of the condition. Topical therapies, such as corticosteroids and calcineurin inhibitors, are commonly prescribed for localised pustular lesions. Systemic medications, including retinoids, methotrexate, cyclosporine, and biologic agents, are reserved for more severe cases or when topical treatments are ine ective. It is essential to monitor patients closely for adverse e ects and adjust treatment regimens as needed to achieve optimal

outcomes. In addition to medical interventions, lifestyle modi cations, stress management techniques, and regular skin care practices can help improve overal wel -being and minimise disease ares.

Prognosis:

The prognosis of pustular psoriasis varies depending on factors such as disease severity, response to treatment, and the presence of comorbidities. With appropriate management, many individuals experience signi cant symptom relief and long-term remission.

However, the chronic nature of the condition necessitates ongoing monitoring and maintenance therapy to prevent relapses and complications. Close col aboration between patients, healthcare providers, and support networks is crucial in managing the physical and emotional aspects of living with pustular psoriasis.

Conclusion:

Pustular psoriasis is a chal enging dermatological condition characterised by the formation of pus- l ed blisters on the skin's surface. While relatively rare compared to other forms of psoriasis, it can have a profound impact on patients' quality of life and requires specialised care. Through a multidisciplinary approach involving dermatologists, rheumatologists, and other healthcare professionals, individuals with pustular psoriasis can receive comprehensive treatment tailored to their needs. By raising awareness, advancing research, and promoting holistic management

strategies, we can strive towards better outcomes and improved wel -being for those a ected by this complex autoimmune disorder.

1.2:(e)Erythrodermic psoriasis:

Erythrodermic psoriasis is an uncommon and severe type of psoriasis. Most of your body is covered with a red, peeling rash. It might be painful and/or itchy. You may feel a burning sensation. The condition is more common in people who already have another type of psoriasis.

Certain medications, like corticosteroids, can trigger it.

So can an injury or severe sunburn. Sometimes, doctors aren't sure what causes it. Erythrodermic psoriasis can lead to other health problems like dehydration, infections, or kidney failure if it's not treated right away. Here's what you need to know.

This is a rare but very dangerous form of psoriasis. It's important to know the symptoms. If you think you have erythrodermic psoriasis, see your doctor right away.Erythrodermic psoriasis is a rare and severe form of psoriasis characterised by widespread in ammation and scaling of the skin. It accounts for only a smal percentage of psoriasis cases, but its e ects can be debilitating and potential y life-threatening if left untreated.

Symptoms:

Fiery red skin from head to toe is the main symptom.

Your skin is also covered in scales and peels o in large

pieces. It can be very painful and itchy. You might see tiny blisters cal ed pustules that are l ed with pus.

Symptoms can develop over time, but they can come on suddenly, too.

You also may have:

- Chil s or a fever

- Joint pain

- A rapid heartbeat

- Swol en ankles

Why It's Dangerous:

Your skin is important to your overal health. It helps control your body temperature, keeps germs and toxins out, and holds moisture in. Erythrodermic psoriasis throws al this o , and the results can be life-threatening. They include a dangerously low body temperature (hypothermia), the loss of much needed proteins and uids, and severe il nesses like sepsis and pneumonia. If you lose too much uid, your heart won't have enough blood to pump. That can lead to shock, kidney failure, and heart failure.

Causes:

The exact cause of erythrodermic psoriasis is not ful y understood, but it is believed to result from a combination of genetic predisposition, immune system dysfunction, and triggers such as infections, withdrawal of systemic corticosteroids. Certain medications, such as lithium, antimalarial drugs, and

beta-blockers, have been associated with triggering or exacerbating erythrodermic psoriasis in susceptible individuals.

Psoriasis is an autoimmune disease. It's when your body's natural defence system attacks healthy tissue.

You're more likely to get erythrodermic psoriasis if you already have plaque psoriasis, especial y if it's unstable.

That means the raised, scaly patches don't have wel -de ned edges. But it also a ects people who've never had the disease.

It can appear if you suddenly stop taking your oral psoriasis medication. Other triggers include:

- Alcoholism

- A drug reaction

- HIV

- An infection

- Oral steroid medicine

- A severe sunburn

● Stress

Diagnosis:

Diagnosing erythrodermic psoriasis typical y involves a thorough physical examination and medical history review by a dermatologist or healthcare provider. The characteristic appearance of widespread erythema and scaling, along with associated symptoms, often points to the diagnosis. In some cases, a skin biopsy may be performed to con rm the diagnosis and rule out other skin conditions with similar presentations.

Your doctor wil start by asking about your health history and doing a physical exam. They'l ask if:

● You have a family history of psoriasis

● You've been exposed to a disease-related trigger like steroids, an infection, or an abrupt stop of psoriasis medicines.

Then they'l check you for signs of psoriasis like:

● Plaques

● Joint pain

● Psoriatic nail disease

They'l probably do a skin biopsy. The doctor wil remove a smal piece of your skin and check it in the lab for signs of

psoriasis.

Treatment Options:

If you have symptoms of erythrodermic psoriasis, don't wait to get help. Go to the hospital right away. Doctors wil try to stop the are-up as quickly as possible and protect you from complications.

Management of erythrodermic psoriasis requires a comprehensive approach aimed at reducing in ammation, control ing symptoms, and preventing complications. Treatment options may include: 1. **Topical Therapies**:

To soothe your skin from the outside, you can use:

● Steroid cream or ointment moisturisers

● Wet wraps

● Oatmeal baths

● Emol ients, moisturisers, and topical corticosteroids may provide symptomatic relief and help restore the skin barrier function.

2. **Systemic Medications**:

Oral medications such as methotrexate, cyclosporine, acitretin, or biologic agents like TNF-alpha inhibitors (e.g., etanercept, adalimumab) may be prescribed to suppress the immune response and reduce skin in ammation.

These medicines are powerful and can have many side e ects. Talk to your doctor to nd out if they're right for you. Make sure they're aware of any other medical conditions you have or any other medications you take.

3. **Phototherapy:** Control ed exposure to ultraviolet (UV) light, either through ultraviolet B (UVB) phototherapy or psoralen plus ultraviolet A (PUVA) therapy, can help al eviate symptoms and promote skin healing.

4. **Supportive Care:** In severe cases, hospitalisation may be necessary to provide supportive care, including intravenous uids, electrolyte replacement, and temperature regulation.

Other treatments.

You may also need:

- Antibiotics to help prevent infection

- Pain medication

- Drugs to control itching

- Medications to relieve anxiety.

Can It Be Prevented?

Some risk factors can't be avoided, like a family history of psoriasis. But you can:

- Let your doctor know if you're having a reaction to a new medication.

- Be careful with anything that could irritate your skin.

- Never abruptly stop taking a psoriasis medication.

- Cover and treat wounds to prevent infection.

- Use phototherapy devices careful y to avoid burns.

- Manage stress.

- Avoid alcohol.

Complications:

Erythrodermic psoriasis can lead to various complications, especial y if left untreated or poorly managed. These may include:

Dehydration and Electrolyte Imbalance: Excessive uid loss through the skin can result in dehydration and electrolyte abnormalities, which may require medical intervention.

Infection:

The compromised skin barrier increases the risk of bacterial, viral, or fungal infections, potential y leading to cel ulitis, sepsis, or pneumonia.

Cardiovascular E ects:

Chronic in ammation associated with psoriasis may contribute to an increased risk of cardiovascular diseases such as heart attack and stroke.

Psychological Impact:

The physical discomfort, dis gurement, and chronic nature of erythrodermic psoriasis can signi cantly impact patients' quality of life, leading to depression, anxiety, and social isolation.

In conclusion

erythrodermic psoriasis is a severe and potential y life-threatening form of psoriasis characterised by widespread in ammation and scaling of the skin. Early diagnosis and prompt initiation of appropriate treatment are essential to al eviate symptoms, prevent complications, and improve patients' overal prognosis and quality of life. A multidisciplinary approach involving dermatologists, primary care physicians, and other healthcare professionals is often necessary to e ectively manage this chal enging condition.

1.3)Causes and Triggers Of Psoriasis: What Causes Psoriasis?

Psoriasis is common. About 2% of people living in the United States have this condition.

Most people who get psoriasis have white skin, but the condition develops in people of al races. Findings from studies indicate that psoriasis may be more common in skin of colour than previously thought. In one US

study, researchers found that 3.6% of whites, nearly 2%

of African Americans, and 1.6% of Hispanics had psoriasis.

Psoriasis runs in families:

If a parent, grandparent, brother, or sister has psoriasis, you have a higher risk of getting it.

Psoriasis is not contagious. Unlike chickenpox or a cold, you cannot catch psoriasis from someone.

You also can not get psoriasis by:

• Swimming in a pool with someone who has psoriasis.

• Touching someone. who has psoriasis.

• Having sex with someone who has psoriasis.

While we know that psoriasis isn't contagious, scientists are stil trying to determine exactly how psoriasis develops.

Scientists have learned that a person's immune system and genes play a role in causing psoriasis. Here's what studies have revealed about each of these.

Immune system:

White blood cel s, also cal ed T-cel s, are part of the body's immune system. These cel s help prevent us from getting sick by attacking things that can harm us, such as bacteria and viruses.

When a person has psoriasis, something goes wrong in the immune system, so T-cel s also attack the body's skin cel s. This attack causes the body to make new skin cel s more often. The extra skin cel s pile up on the surface of the skin, and you see psoriasis.

Once T-cel s start to attack skin cel s, this usual y continues for the rest of a person's life. There is one exception. Some children who get a type of psoriasis cal ed guttate (gut-tate) psoriasis never have it again.

Genes:

We know that psoriasis runs in families. Scientists have found that people who have certain genes are more likely to get psoriasis.

What complicates matters is what else scientists have learned. It seems that some people who get psoriasis don't have genes that increase their risk of getting psoriasis.

It's also possible to have genes that increase the risk of getting psoriasis and never develop psoriasis. It's this discovery that led

Scientists believe that the person must be exposed to a trigger before psoriasis appears.

What Triggers Psoriasis Flare-ups?

If your psoriasis seems to are for no reason, one or more triggers could be to blame. Everyday things like stress, a bug bite, and cold temperatures can trigger psoriasis.

By nding your triggers and learning how to manage them, you can gain better control of your psoriasis and have fewer ares.

To nd yours, you'l have to do a bit of detective work.

A good place to start is by looking at this chart of the common triggers, which also gives you signs that it could be a trigger for you.

There is a wide range of factors that can impact when and where your psoriasis symptoms appear, reappear, or even worsen. On top of that, these triggers can vary from person to person, so it's important to know what your speci c triggers are.While the underlying cause of psoriasis stems from your body's immune system, certain triggers can make symptoms worse or cause are-ups.

Here are a few common psoriasis triggers: **i)Stress:**

Having psoriasis can itself cause stress, and patients often report that outbreaks of symptoms come during particularly stressful times.For those with psoriasis, stress can sometimes trigger in ammation and may

cause symptoms to appear, reappear, or even worsen.Stress is a common trigger.

Reduce risk of are-ups from stress:

● Find a way to manage your stress and practise it

— even when you're feeling okay. Common stress busters include yoga, meditation, and support groups.

● Before going to sleep, write down 3 things that you're grateful for. Do this daily.

- When you start to feel stressed, take a deep breath, hold it, and exhale slowly.

ii)Skin Injury:

Scratches,Bumps,and Bruises, al can irritate your skin and kick your immune system into high gear, aggravating your psoriasis.

If this triggers your psoriasis, you'l get a are-up near (or in the same spot as) the injury or bite. This happens about 10 to 14 days after you injure your skin.

Flare-ups happen after getting a cut, scrape, sunburn, scratch, outbreak of poison ivy, bruise, or bug bite.

Reduce the risk of are-ups from a skin injury:

- If you injure your skin, treat it quickly.

- If your skin itches, calm the itch.

- Avoid scratching, which can trigger a are.

- Try to avoid getting bug bites by using insect repel ent and staying indoors

when bugs are most active. Bugs are most active at dusk and dawn.

iii)Smoking;

Does your psoriasis are unexpectedly? If you smoke or spend time with people who smoke, this could be the cause.

Reduce the risk of are-ups from drinking:

- Stop smoking. Because this can be di cult, ask your dermatologist or primary care doctor for help.

- Before trying a nicotine patch, ask your dermatologist whether using it could trigger your psoriasis.

• Avoid being around people who are smoking.

iv)Cold and dry weather:

General y, fal and winter are worse for your psoriasis than warmer seasons. A combination of dry air, less sunlight, and colder temperatures can contribute to cold-weather are-ups.

Such weather can dry out your skin, which makes the chances of having a are-up worse. In contrast, hot, sunny weather appears to help control the symptoms of psoriasis in most people.

Reduce the risk of are-ups from dry, cold weather:

• Treat your psoriasis.

• Limit showers and baths to 10 minutes and use warm rather than hot water.

• Immediately after bathing, slather on moisturiser, using a fragrance-free ointment or cream rather than a lotion.

• Use a gentle, moisturising cleanser instead of soap.

• Apply moisturiser throughout the day when your skin feels dry.

• Plug in a humidi er when the air in your home feels dry.

• Stay warm and protect your skin from extreme weather when outside by wearing a hat, gloves, waterproof boots, and a winter jacket.

• Sit far enough away from a replace, radiator, or other heat source so that you cannot feel the heat on your skin.

• Remove wet clothes and footwear when you come in from the cold.

v)Sunshine, warm weather;

During warm weather, psoriasis can are if you:

- Sunburn

- Spend time in air conditioning.

Reduce the risk of are-ups during warm weather

- If you spend time in air conditioning, apply moisturiser immediately after showering or getting out of a bath.

- If your skin stil feels dry from spending time in air conditioning, apply moisturiser throughout the day.

- Avoid sunburn by wearing sunscreen. You want to apply sunscreen to skin that clothing doesn't cover and is free of psoriasis. To get the protection you need, use sunscreen that o ers broad-spectrum protection, SPF 30 or higher, and water resistance.

vi)Infection:

One of your immune system's major roles is ghting infection. For those with psoriasis, the body's overactive immune system can send faulty signals that in turn trigger in ammation to continue even after the infection has been cleared.

Psoriasis can are 2 to 6 weeks after strep throat, an earache, bronchitis, or another infection. This is especial y common in kids.

Reduce the risk of are-ups due to infection: Treat the infection. This can lessen or clear the psoriasis.

Tel your dermatologist if you have an HIV (human immunode ciency virus) infection, which can make some psoriasis treatments risky.

vii)Medication

Some medications can cause a are-up. If a medication is a trigger for you, you'l are 2 to 3 weeks after beginning a medication.

Reduce the risk of are-ups from medication: If you think a medication is causing your psoriasis to are, don,t stop taking it. Ask the doctor who prescribed it whether the medicine could be causing your psoriasis to are. If it could, ask if you could take another medication.

Before taking a medicine for the rst time, ask the doctor prescribing it if the medicine could cause psoriasis to are. Medicines that commonly trigger psoriasis include lithium, drugs taken to prevent malaria, strong corticosteroids like prednisone (if you quit taking it rapidly instead of stepping down), medicine that treats high blood pressure and problems with your heartbeat, and some arthritis medications.

viii)Shaving:

If you cut yourself while shaving, you may notice new psoriasis about 10 to 14 days later where you cut yourself.

Reduce your risk of are-ups from shaving:

- Take care to avoid cutting yourself while shaving.

- **Dermatologists' tip:** To reduce cuts and nicks, try applying moisturiser and then shaving gel before you shave.

ix)Drinking frequently or in excess: If you drink daily or have more than 2 drinks in a day frequently, your treatment for psoriasis may have little or no e ect. Even treatment that could be e ective for you may not work and you'l continue to have are-ups.

Reduce the risk of are-ups from drinking:

- Quit drinking.

- If you continue to drink, limit how much you drink in a day. Women should stop after 1

drink. Men should limit themselves to 2 drinks per day.

• Be sure to tel your dermatologist if you drink alcohol. Drinking can make it risky to take some psoriasis medications like methotrexate.

Chapter-(2)

Diagnosis and Symptoms of psoriasis: 2.1:Recognizing Psoriasis Symptoms.

2.2)Seeking Medical Diagnosis.

2.1:Recognizing Psoriasis Symptoms.

The signs and symptoms of psoriasis depend on the type of psoriasis and factors speci c to each person.

Some people with one type of psoriasis may go on to develop an additional type.

Psoriasis is an autoimmune condition that causes skin symptoms.Skin changes can look di erent on di erent people.

The a ected areas may be pink, coral, or red, especial y on light skin. On skin of colour, the areas may instead be purple, violet, or grey. Or they may be the same colour as the surrounding skin, making the changes more di cult to see. This can contribute to chal enges and inequities in diagnosis and treatment.

Most people with psoriasis have ares and periods of remission, where symptoms may lessen or go away.

During a are, the symptoms worsen for a while. There is currently no cure for psoriasis, but treatment can lead to remission for a prolonged time.After years of living with psoriasis, some people may develop other types of psoriasis.

Below,are the symptoms of psoriasis as per their types:-

Plaque psoriasis symptoms:

Plaque Psoriasis is the most common type of psoriasis.

A person with plaque psoriasis may experience these changes:

• Raised, in amed lesions, cal ed plaques, develop. These are often covered in a silvery white scale.

• The plaques can develop anywhere but are more common on the elbows, scalp, knees, and lower back.

• The plaques may join together.

• They may be itchy, sore, or both.

• Psoriasis lesions on the skin around the joints may crack and bleed.

• On lighter skin tones, plaque psoriasis usual y appears as pink or red patches with silvery white scales. On skin of colour, psoriasis may form purplish or brown patches with grey scales.

Inverse Psoriasis symptoms:

Inverse psoriasis tends to appear in skin folds, and it is more common among people who are overweight.

A person with the condition may nd that:

• Patches of skin become in amed and smooth, but there is no scaling.

• These patches become itchy or painful.

• Symptoms can worsen if the skin rubs together or sweating in the folds occurs.

• It is most likely to develop in the armpits, groynes, between the buttocks, beneath the breasts, and bel y folds if a person has these.

• On brown or darker skin, the lesions may be purple, brown, or a darker colour than the surrounding skin. On lighter skin tones, they may be bright red.

According to research published in 2016 suggests that 21–30% of people with psoriasis develop inverse psoriasis.

Nail Psoriasis Symptoms:

Nail psoriasis can a ect the ngernails and toenails. It may develop with another type of psoriasis.

Severe symptoms can make it hard to use the hands and feet as per my own personal experience.

Here are some of the features of nail psoriasis:

• white, yel ow, or brown discoloration that may resemble a drop of oil or blood under the nail plate

• pits in the nails

• lines across the nails, either from side to side rather than top to bottom

• light areas on the nail plate

• thickening of the skin under the nail

• loosening, separating, lifting, and detaching of the nail

• crumbling, as the nail weakens

• smal black lines running from the tip of the nail to the cuticle

• spotting or reddening of the "half moon" at the base of the nail

• possibly, an infection in the area

• blood under the nail plate

• Nail changes can also be a sign of a type of arthritis cal ed psoriatic arthritis. If a person notices nail changes, they may need to talk with a doctor.

Guttate Psoriasis symptoms:

Guttate psoriasis is sometimes known as "tear drop" or "raindrop" psoriasis.

Here are some of the features:

• Lesions usual y appear quickly, within a few days.

• The lesions are smal , round spots, or papules — unlike plaque psoriasis.

• They often develop on the arms, legs, and trunk, but they may form on the face, ears, and scalp, too.

• The papules do not hurt but may itch.

• Guttate psoriasis can occur after tonsilitis, strep throat, or another infection. A skin injury or stress may also trigger it. Research published in 2009 suggests that around 8% of people with psoriasis wil develop guttate

psoriasis at some time.

Pustular Psoriasis Symptoms:

Pustular psoriasis is less common than other forms of psoriasis. There are di erent types of pustular psoriasis, depending on what area of the body is a ected.

Below are some common features:

• Reddish pus- l ed bumps appear.

• Pustules can develop anywhere on the skin, including in the mouth or under a nail.

- They tend to join together and burst around 24–48 hours after they form.

- As pus dries, the skin becomes glazed and often painful.

- New pustules can form in the same area, and the cycle of joining and bursting can repeat.

- If these pustules a ect widespread areas of the body, the person needs immediate medical attention to prevent life threatening complications.

Erythrodermic Psoriasis Symptoms: Erythrodermic psoriasis is the least common type. It can be life threatening without treatment.

The symptoms include:

- widespread in ammation

- severe discoloration of the skin, such as redness

- a burned appearance to the skin

- intense itching and pain

- shedding of skin in large sheets rather than smal er scales

- As the skin becomes damaged, it loses its barrier function, which means that the skin is less able to protect the body. The person's temperature may uctuate, and they may start to lose proteins and uid. This can lead to dehydration and heart failure.

Other symptoms include:

- chil s, a fever, and a general feeling of being unwel

- muscle weakness

- a rapid pulse

- swel ing (edema), especial y in the lower legs

● Anyone with a painful, widespread rash needs urgent medical treatment.

2.2)Seeking Medical Diagnosis:

Psoriasis is an autoimmune disease that causes skin cel s to multiply up to 10 times faster than normal. There is a wide spectrum of severity and manifestations of psoriasis, but common characteristics of most types of psoriasis include skin redness (erythema), thickening, and scaling (squamae).

General y, psoriasis causes tel tale patches of thick, red, scaly skin that can be spotted during a physical exam.

Sometimes this is enough to diagnose psoriasis.

However, when the diagnosis is uncertain, a provider may also perform a skin biopsy to col ect tissue samples that can be examined under a microscope.

In most cases, your primary care doctor or dermatologist wil be able to diagnose psoriasis by examining your skin. However, since psoriasis can look like eczema and other skin diseases, diagnosing it can sometimes be di cult.

If your doctor isn't sure whether you have psoriasis, they may order a biopsy. Your doctor wil remove a smal sample of your skin and have it looked at under a microscope.

If you have symptoms of psoriatic arthritis, such as swol en and painful joints, your doctor might run

blood tests and take X-rays to rule out other forms of arthritis.

Diagnostic process:

Diagnosing psoriasis typical y involves a comprehensive evaluation of the patient's medical history, physical examination, and sometimes, additional tests. The diagnosis of psoriasis is primarily made through clinical examination. However, in some cases, a skin biopsy or other medical tests may aid in the diagnosis.

Key diagnostic criteria include:

Clinical examination:

A medical history and physical examination are the most common diagnostic tools used for psoriasis.

Clinical clues that suggest psoriasis include the fol owing:

a)Physical Examination:

The diagnosis of psoriasis is usual y made upon physical examination, fol owing a discussion about the family and medical history of the patient.

There are many health conditions that can cause itchy, scaly skin and rashes. In most cases, healthcare practitioners—especial y dermatologists, who specialise in skin disorders—can tel if your symptoms are due to psoriasis or something else based on sight alone.

To get a closer look, they may view your skin through a dermatoscope. This simple handheld tool has a light

and a magnifying glass. It al ows your doctor to "zoom in" on your skin

b)Review of Medical History:

It is important to discuss the family and medical history when a patient is suspected to be experiencing symptoms of psoriasis. This is because there is a strong hereditary link with psoriasis and approximately one-third of people with psoriasis have a close family member with the condition.

There are several types of psoriasis. Some can cause symptoms that a ect more than your skin, so your practitioner may ask if anything else is bothering you too.

In addition, they wil likely ask you if you have any other risk factors for psoriasis, such as:

- A family history of psoriasis or other skin conditions

- A recent strep throat infection

- A recent vaccine

- A condition that weakens your immune system, like HIV

- Other autoimmune disorders, such as celiac disease, Crohn's disease, or thyroid disease.

c)Skin examination:

The diagnosis of psoriasis is primarily conducted with an examination of the skin, based on the appearance of the skin and the reported symptoms of the patient.

The a ected area can be visual y examined for signs of psoriasis on the skin, such as red patches and scaliness on the top. The speci c symptoms depend on the type of psoriasis, but the general signs may include:

- Redness

- Scaliness

- Plaque

- Skin lesions

- Nail changes

- Itching

- In ammation

- Pain

Skin biopsy;

A sample of skin may be biopsied for examination under a microscope. A biopsy is usual y reserved for atypical presentations of psoriasis or to exclude other disorders, such as eczema or skin infections. Common types of skin biopsies include the fol owing:
Punch biopsy

A punch biopsy involves the use of a round, circular tool (similar to a paper-hole punch) to remove a smal core of skin.

Shave biopsy

A shave biopsy involves the use of a blade to cut o the outermost layer of skin.

Excisional biopsy

An excisional biopsy involves the removal of an entire lesion on the skin and, in some cases, requires a skin graft to repair the area.

Incisional biopsy

An incisional biopsy involves the removal of a section of a large lesion.A positive skin biopsy for psoriasis may show a large number of activated T cel s; the absence of normal cel maturation; or an increased number of basal cel s (known as basal cel hyperplasia). Basal cel s produce new skin cel s.

d)Other laboratory tests and studies While additional labs, tests and studies are not usual y needed to diagnose psoriasis, any of the fol owing may be ordered:

Fungal studies

Fungal studies may be ordered to rule out fungal infections.

Erythrocyte sedimentation rate (ESR) An ESR blood test may be ordered to check for systemic in ammation. ESR may be elevated with pustular or erythrodermic psoriasis.

Autoantibody studies.

When psoriatic arthritis is suspected, autoantibody tests may be ordered to rule out other types of arthritis.

These tests may include a rheumatoid factor (RF)

blood test, which may indicate rheumatoid arthritis; or an antinuclear antibody (ANA) test, which may indicate lupus.

Imaging studies

Images from X-rays and bone scans can aid in the diagnosis of psoriatic arthritis.

Baseline laboratory studies

Baseline laboratory studies may be ordered when starting systemic therapies, such as biologics.

Laboratory tests may include a complete blood count (CBC), complete metabolic panel (CMP), hepatitis panel, tuberculosis screening, or pregnancy test.

Chapter-(3)

Treatment Options:

3.1:Topical Treatments.

3.2:Phototherapy.

3.3:Oral Medications.

3.4:Biologics treatment options.

3.5:Prevention of Psoriasis.

Psoriasis treatment aims to al eviate symptoms, reduce in ammation, and prevent complications. Treatment options vary depending on the severity of the condition and may include:

3.1:Topical Treatments Of Psoriasis: Based on the appearance of your skin, your doctor determines if one or a combination of topical medications is right for you. Topical medication is usual y most e ective for people with mild to moderate

psoriasis, meaning lesions cover less than 10 percent of their bodies.

If topical medication relieves your symptoms, your doctor may recommend you use it for years, as part of a long-term treatment plan. Throughout treatment, he or she monitors how wel the medication is working during periodic fol ow-up visits. Your doctor also looks for any side e ects, such as thinning skin at the site of application. If you have side e ects, your doctor may adjust how often you apply the medication or prescribe a di erent type.

Topical medication may lead to dry skin, which can exacerbate psoriasis symptoms. Doctors often recommend using an over-the-counter moisturiser, as wel .

Corticosteroids;

Corticosteroids are prescription medications that reduce in ammation, which causes itching, swel ing, and redness. They also prevent the body from overproducing new skin cel s and slow the formation of new lesions.

Corticosteroid creams and gels are available in varying potencies. Your dermatologist may recommend a low potency for sensitive areas of skin, such as the face and genitals, and a higher potency for very thick lesions or those that don't respond to less potent forms.

Corticosteroid shampoos are available for people with scalp psoriasis or dandru .

The side e ects associated with long-term use of topical corticosteroids include thinning skin and discoloration.

Your dermatologist determines how long you should use topical steroids and may recommend other forms of treatment for long-term use.

Vitamin D Analogues;

Topical medication chemical y related to but distinct from vitamin D inhibits the growth of skin cel s and may reduce the number of new psoriasis lesions. Your dermatologist may recommend this medication in addition to other forms of treatment, such as light therapy, to enhance their e ectiveness.

Coal Tar;

Coal tar is a substance derived from coal that can slow skin cel growth and reduce the redness, swel ing, and itching of psoriasis. This medication is available over the counter or by prescription as a cream, ointment, foam, or shampoo.

Some people nd topical coal tar medication e ective, but it may leave a dark stain on clothing or bedding.

Medication with coal tar also makes the skin more sensitive to sun exposure; doctors recommend you

apply a broad-spectrum sunscreen of SPF 30 or higher whenever you spend time in the sun.

Salicylic Acid;

Salicylic acid is an ingredient in many over-the-counter and prescription creams, gels, and shampoos used to treat psoriasis. It may improve the appearance of skin by removing dead skin cel s, including the white or silver scales of plaques.

Anthralin;

Anthralin is a synthetic form of a natural substance found in the bark of the South American araroba tree.

When applied as a topical medication, anthralin slows the growth of skin cel s. Your dermatologist may recommend this medication when psoriasis is resistant to other topical treatments. Anthralin may be used in combination with another topical therapy, such as corticosteroids.

Anthralin is available by prescription in varying strengths. Your doctor determines which strength is right for you based on the appearance of your skin and other symptoms.

Calcineurin Inhibitors;

Your doctor may recommend a calcineurin inhibitor if psoriasis a ects sensitive areas of the body, such as eyelids or genitals. The medication blocks calcineurin, a protein that plays a role in skin in ammation.

Retinoids;

Your doctor may recommend a topical retinoid cream or gel to improve the appearance of psoriasis, including thickened ngernails and toenails. Retinoids, derived from vitamin A, reduce in ammation and slow down cel turnover—the rate at which new cel s replace old ones—helping nails remain healthy and appear less chalky and thick.

3.2:Phototherapy Treatment For Psoriasis: If the medicine you put on your skin isn't doing al that it needs to, your doctor may suggest adding phototherapy to your psoriasis treatment. It uses ultraviolet rays that come from sunshine, arti cial lamps, or lasers to slow skin cel growth and ease your symptoms.

While dermatologists prescribe phototherapy for many people, it is not recommended for anyone who has:

• Had a melanoma or any other type of skin cancer

• A medical condition that makes you more likely to develop skin cancer, such as Gorlin syndrome or xeroderma .

• A medical condition that makes you sensitive to UV light, such as lupus or porphyria

• To take medicine that makes them more sensitive to UV light, such as some antibiotics, diuretics, and antifungals.

How to use

Phototherapy is usual y given at a psoriasis treatment centre or hospital. To be e ective, most patients need two or three phototherapy treatments a week. This means that you must go to the treatment centre or hospital two or three times a week for several weeks. In some cases, you may need to go ve times a week.

There are di erent types of phototherapy. The most common types that dermatologists prescribe are: **Types of Phototherapy:**

Sunlight.

Too many rays coming directly from the sun can make your symptoms worse and raise your chances of getting skin cancer. If your doctor tel s you to get some sun each day, about 20 minutes a day should be enough.

Use a sunscreen with zinc oxide and an SPF of 30 or higher on areas of your skin that don't have psoriasis.

UVB (ultraviolet B).

Your doctor can treat you with UVB rays from a phototherapy machine in their o ce. You can also get one to use at home. But the lamps can give o ultraviolet A (UVA) rays. Both UVA and UVB rays are linked to skin cancer. Talk to your doctor about how to

protect yourself from the cancer risk while being treated.

There are 2 main types of UVB treatments: **UVB broadband:**

Your health care provider may use it to treat single patches, widespread psoriasis, and psoriasis that doesn't improve with topical treatments. In the short term, side e ects might include redness, itching, and dry skin.

Moisturising regularly can help ease your discomfort.

UVB narrowband: Many scientists and doctors think this type of UVB is more e ective than broadband. But you may notice more serious burns from the treatments that last longer. Narrowband UVB light bulbs release a smal er range of ultraviolet light. The treatment seems to work more quickly and keep psoriasis ares away for longer. And it often requires fewer treatments per week.

PUVA (psoralen plus ultraviolet A).

This treatment combines UVA lamp sessions with a drug cal ed psoralen. You either take the drug as a pil or put it on your skin as a cream, lotion, gel, solution, or ointment. It makes your skin more sensitive to light.

The process is cal ed photochemotherapy. You'l probably go to your doctor's o ce 2 or 3 times a week for a total of 25 to 30 sessions.

PUVA clears up psoriasis quickly with long-lasting results. But using it for a long time can raise your

chances of skin cancer. Because of that, it's typical y only recommended for severe cases or when other treatments haven't worked.

The treatment also has side e ects such as:

- Nausea

- Exhaustion

- Headaches

- Burning and itching

Because psoralen makes your body extra sensitive to light, you need to protect your skin and eyes after taking it. Wear glasses that block ultraviolet light, and wear sunscreen for at least the rst 24 hours after treatment.

Lasers.

These highly focused beams of light target your psoriasis patches, not your healthy skin. This cuts down on side e ects and may lower your chances of skin cancer. You'l also need fewer treatments compared with other types of light therapy.

The excimer laser uses focused, high-energy ultraviolet B light. It can help patches get better faster than other methods. You usual y get this treatment in your doctor's o ce twice a week for 4 or 5 weeks.

Doctors also sometimes use pulsed dye lasers, or PDLs, to treat psoriasis. PDLs use a liquid with an organic dye to create a laser that delivers gentle bursts of focused light onto careful y targeted areas of skin. The heat that

results clears away damaged blood vessels but keeps surrounding skin as safe as possible.

Side e ects from laser therapy are general y mild, but some people say it can hurt a bit. You may also have bruising, sunburns, and possibly scarring at the spots that have been treated.

After laser treatment, you should stay out of sunlight and be careful not to injure the area. Cal your doctor if you see blisters.

Home UVB phototherapy.

There are units available for home use to deliver UVB

phototherapy. As with al phototherapy treatments, these require a doctor's prescription. When you use it, you need to keep a consistent treatment schedule as instructed by your doctor. Ask your doctor if you are a good candidate for one of these units.

Grenz rays. This approach is less common. Doctors give this treatment with "super cial X-ray machines" to deliver a form of soft X-rays that work in a way similar to UV light.

Photodynamic therapy. Though not common, your doctor may suggest photodynamic therapy for your psoriasis. This procedure uses special medicines that intensify the e ects of a light source. Side e ects of burned skin can limit the usefulness of this approach in

the treatment of psoriasis. But scientists continue to study new versions of this treatment in search of better results.

Why do dermatologists prescribe phototherapy for psoriasis?

This treatment can:

- Slow rapidly growing skin cel s

- Suppress an overly active immune system

- Reduce in ammation and al ow the skin to heal

- Reduce or eliminate the itch

Safety and e ectiveness

Most people who have psoriasis can use a type of phototherapy cal ed narrowband UVB. Dermatologists prescribe this for children, women who are pregnant or breastfeeding, and people who have a weakened immune system or an ongoing infection. The excimer laser provides a type of narrowband UVB

phototherapy that can safely treat children and adults who have psoriasis on the scalp, ears, armpits, groyne, or buttocks. This laser can also safely treat areas like the elbows and knees.

SALICYLIC ACID WARNING

Going for phototherapy treatment? Don't apply your salicylic acid (used to treat acne and psoriasis scale) beforehand. When applied to the skin before phototherapy, salicylic acid can make

UVB phototherapy less effective.

Research shows that di erent types of phototherapy can e ectively treat:

• Smal areas of stubborn, thick plaque psoriasis

• Palmoplantar (on hands and feet) psoriasis that you've had for a long time

• Plaque psoriasis that covers a large amount of skin

• Nail psoriasis

• Scalp psoriasis

Possible side e ects:

While phototherapy is considered safe, medical treatments carry possible side e ects. With phototherapy, the possible side e ects that can happen immediately after treatment include:

• Sunburn-like reaction (red or tender skin)

• Mild stinging or burning

• Dark spots on the skin (more common in people who have a medium to dark

complexion)

• Itching

• Blisters (rare)

• Burn (rare)

• After each treatment, your skin should be a little red or pink. This is desirable and not considered a side e ect.

Possible long-term side e ects include:

- Freckles

- Early skin ageing (age spots, wrinkles, loose skin)

- Increased risk of developing skin cancer Under a dermatologist's care, these long-term side e ects can be managed.

What to discuss with your dermatologist: If you use phototherapy to treat psoriasis, your dermatologist wil check you after you have had a certain number of treatments, usual y four to six in the beginning. These checkups are essential, so be sure to keep al of your appointments.

During these appointments with your dermatologist, you should tel your dermatologist if you have:

- Any side e ects

- Worsening psoriasis after phototherapy

- Missed more than two appointments If you miss appointments, it's unlikely that phototherapy wil be helpful for you. Research shows that patients see steady improvement only when they receive phototherapy two to ve times per week.

3.3:Systemics or Oral Medication options for psoriasis:

Psoriasis is a common autoimmune disorder that causes red, thick, in amed patches of skin. The patches are often covered in whitish silvery scales cal ed plaques. In some cases, the a ected skin wil crack, bleed, or ooze. Many people feel burning, pain, and tenderness around the a ected skin. Psoriasis is a chronic condition. Even with treatment, psoriasis wil never ful y go away. Therefore, treatment aims to reduce symptoms and to help the disease enter remission. Remission is a period of little to no disease activity. This means there are fewer symptoms. There are a range of treatment options available for psoriasis, including oral medications. Oral drugs are a form of systemic treatment, which means they a ect your whole body. These drugs can be very strong, so doctors typical y only prescribe them for severe psoriasis. In many cases, these drugs are reserved for people who haven't had much success with other psoriasis treatments. Unfortunately, they can cause a variety of side e ects and issues.Below mentioned are some of the oral treatments for psoriasis:

Option #1: Acitretin:

Acitretin (Soriatane) is an oral retinoid. Retinoids are a form of vitamin A. Acitretin is the only oral retinoid used to treat severe psoriasis in adults. It can cause serious side e ects. Because of this, your doctor may only prescribe this medication for a short time. When

your psoriasis enters remission, your doctor may advise you to stop taking this drug until you have another are-up.

Side e ects of acitretin

The more common side e ects of acitretin include:

- chapped skin and lips

- hair loss

- dry mouth

- aggressive thoughts

- changes in your mood and behaviour

- depression

- headache

- pain behind your eyes

- joint pain

- liver damage

In rare cases, serious side e ects can occur. Cal your doctor right away if you experience any of the fol owing:

- a change in vision or a loss of night vision

- bad headaches

- nausea

- shortness of breath

- swel ing

- chest pain

- weakness

- trouble speaking

- yel owing of your skin or the whites of your eyes

Option #2: Cyclosporine:

Cyclosporine is an immunosuppressant. It's available as the brand-name medications Neoral, Gengraf, and Sandimmune. It's used to treat severe psoriasis if other treatments don't work. Cyclosporine works by calming the immune system. It prevents or stops the overreaction in the body that causes symptoms of psoriasis. This drug is very strong and can cause serious side e ects.

Side e ects of cyclosporine;

The more common side e ects of cyclosporine include:

- headache

- fever

- stomach pain

- nausea

- vomiting

- unwanted hair growth

- diarrhoea

- shortness of breath

- slow or fast heart rate

- changes in urine

- back pain

- swel ing of your hands and feet

- unusual bruising or bleeding

- excessive tiredness

- excessive weakness

- increased blood pressure

- shaky hands (tremor).

Other risks of cyclosporine;

Cyclosporine can cause other problems as wel . These include:

Drug interactions. Some versions of cyclosporine can't be used at the same time or after other psoriasis treatments. Tel your doctor about every drug or treatment you've ever taken and are currently taking.

This includes medications to treat psoriasis, as wel as treatments for other conditions. If you have trouble remembering which drugs you've taken, which many people do, ask your pharmacist for a list of those medications.

Kidney damage.

Your doctor wil check your blood pressure before and during your treatment with this drug. You'l likely also need to have regular urine tests. This is so your doctor can check for possible kidney damage. Your doctor may pause or stop your treatment with cyclosporine to protect your kidneys.

Infections.

Cyclosporine raises your risk of infections. You should avoid being around sick people so you don't pick up their germs. Wash your hands often. If you have signs of an infection, cal your doctor right away.

Nervous system problems.

This drug can also cause nervous system problems. Tel your doctor right away if you have any of these symptoms:

- mental changes

- muscle weakness

- vision changes

- dizziness

- a loss of consciousness

- seizures

- yel owing of your skin or the whites of your eyes

- blood in your urine

Option #3: Methotrexate:

Methotrexate (Trexal) belongs to a drug class cal ed antimetabolites. This drug is given to people with severe psoriasis who have not had much success with other treatments. It can slow the growth of skin cel s and stop scales from forming.

Side e ects of methotrexate:

The more common side e ects of methotrexate include:

- tiredness

- chil s

- fever

- nausea

- stomach pain

- dizziness

- hair loss

- eye redness

- headaches

- tender gums

- loss of appetite

- infections

Your doctor may recommend a folic acid (vitamin B) supplement to help protect against some of these side e ects. In rare cases, this medication can cause serious, life-threatening side e ects. The risk of having these side e ects increases with higher doses of the medication. Cal your doctor right away if you experience any of the fol owing:

- unusual bleeding

- yel owing of your skin or whites of your eyes

- dark-coloured urine or blood in your urine

- dry cough that doesn't produce phlegm

- al ergic reactions, which may include trouble breathing, rash, or hives.

Other risks of methotrexate;

Methotrexate can cause other problems as wel . These include:

● **Drug interactions.**

You shouldn't combine this drug with certain other drugs due to the risk of serious side e ects. These may include anti-in ammatory drugs that are available over the counter. Talk to your doctor about other serious interactions that could occur if you take certain medications.

● **Liver damage**.

If this drug is taken for a long time, it can cause liver damage. You shouldn't take methotrexate if you have liver damage or a history of alcohol abuse or alcoholic liver disease. Your doctor may recommend a liver biopsy to check for liver damage.

● **E ects with kidney disease**.

Talk to your doctor before taking this drug if you have kidney disease. You may need a di erent dosage.

● **Harm to pregnancy.**

Women who are pregnant, breastfeeding, or planning to become pregnant shouldn't use this drug. Men should not get a woman pregnant during treatment and for three months after stopping this drug. Men should use condoms throughout this time.

Option #4: Apremilast:

In 2014, the U.S. Food and Drug Administration (FDA) approved apremilast (Otezla) to treat psoriasis and psoriatic arthritis in adults. Apremilast is thought to work within your immune system and decrease your body's response to in ammation.

Side e ects of apremilast:

According to the FDA, the more common side e ects people experienced during clinical trials included:

- headache

- nausea

- diarrhoea

- vomiting

- cold symptoms, such as a runny nose

- stomach pain

People who were taking this drug also reported depression more frequently during clinical trials than people taking a placebo.

Other risks of apremilast;

Other possible concerns related to the use of apremilast include:

- **Weight loss.**

Apremilast can also cause unexplained weight loss.

Your doctor should monitor your weight for unexplained weight loss during treatment.

- **E ects with kidney**

disease.

Talk to your doctor before taking this drug if you have kidney disease. You may need a di erent dosage.

- **Drug interactions**.

You shouldn't combine apremilast with some other drugs, because they make apremilast less e ective.

Examples of these drugs include the seizure medications carbamazepine, phenytoin, and phenobarbital. Talk to your doctor about other medications you're taking before you start apremilast

3.4:Biologics Treatment option for psoriasis: Biologic drugs, or biologics, are given by injection (shot) or intravenous (IV) infusion (a slow drip of medicine into your vein). A biologic is a protein-based drug derived from living cel s cultured in a laboratory.

While biologics, such as vaccines and insulin, have been used to treat disease for more than 100 years, modern-day techniques have made biologics a viable treatment option for psoriasis in the past 15 years.

Biologics are newer, stronger medicines. A biologic can target, or quiet, only the part of the immune system

that is overactive because of psoriasis. This means that biologics have less risk of causing problems with the liver, kidneys, and other organs than do other strong psoriasis medicines.

Why do dermatologists prescribe a biologic to treat psoriasis?

A biologic is an important treatment option for people with moderate-to-severe psoriasis, psoriatic arthritis, or both. For many people, taking a biologic was life changing because it helped control their symptoms when other treatments failed.

Biologics work by blocking reactions in your body that cause psoriasis and its symptoms. If you have psoriatic arthritis, a biologic can stop the pain, sti ness, and swel ing in your joints. It can prevent the arthritis from worsening and causing more damage to your joints.

The US Food and Drug Administration (FDA) has approved the fol owing biologics to treat adults with psoriasis or psoriatic arthritis. In many cases, these biologics have been approved to treat both diseases.

- Cimzia® (certolizumab pegol)

- Cosentyx® (secukinumab)

- Enbrel® (etanercept)

- Humira® (adalimumab)

- Ilumia™ (til daclizumab)

- Remicade® (in iximab)

- Simponi® (golimumab)

- Skyrizi™ (risankizumab)

- Stelara® (ustekinumab)

- Taltz® (ixekizumab)

- Tremfya™ (guselkumab).

Sometimes, a biologic is prescribed to treat a child who has psoriasis. This can be very e ective for a child who has moderate or severe psoriasis. The FDA has approved the fol owing biologics for children who have moderate or severe psoriasis:

- Etanercept: Approved for children of 4 years of age and older.

- Ustekinumab: Approved for children of 12

years of age and older

- Secukinumab: Approved for children of 6 years of age and older.

Safety and e ectiveness:

Safety:

Overal , biologics have a good safety record.

A patient's risk of developing a serious infection remains the biggest concern. For this reason, dermatologists careful y screen each patient before prescribing a biologic.

You'l need to have some medical tests before your dermatologist can tel whether a biologic can be prescribed to treat your psoriasis. Blood tests and tuberculosis (TB) testing are typical y required. Some patients need additional medical tests.

E ectiveness: Studies show that the biologics approved to treat psoriasis and psoriatic arthritis can be very e ective. For many people with moderate-to-severe psoriasis or psoriatic arthritis, a biologic may o er the most e ective treatment available.

If you take a biologic continuously, it tends to be more e ective. Stopping and starting can cause a biologic to lose its e ectiveness and may cause certain side e ects.

It's also possible for a biologic to stop working after a person takes it for some time. If this happens, another biologic may work.

While a biologic can lose its e ectiveness over time, studies show that for many people a biologic remains an e ective and safe treatment for years.

How to use:

This varies with the type of biologic. You'l either get a shot or an infusion (through an IV). Some shots you can give yourself at home, after learning how to give yourself the shot. In iximab requires an infusion (through an IV), so you'l need to go to your doctor's o ce or an infusion centre for treatment.

How often you take the biologic varies from twice a week to once every three months. Your dermatologist wil tel you how often you should take it.

Possible side e ects:

Each biologic has its own list of possible side e ects.

Most are mild and do not cause patients to stop taking the biologic. Some of the more common side e ects include:

- Upper respiratory tract infection

- Skin reaction where the biologic is injected

- Flu-like symptoms

- Urinary tract infection

- Headache

Because the biologics work by calming down part of your immune system, anyone taking a biologic has an increased risk of developing a serious infection. The risk is higher in patients who have diabetes, smoke or chew tobacco, or have a history of infections. Older patients also have a higher risk.

3.5:Prevention of Psoriasis:

While the exact cause of psoriasis remains unknown, several strategies can help prevent are-ups and manage symptoms e ectively:

1. **Avoid Triggers:** Identify and avoid triggers that exacerbate psoriasis symptoms, such as stress, certain medications, infections, and cold weather.

2. **Maintain a Healthy Lifestyle:** Adopting a balanced diet, regular exercise routine, and adequate sleep can help strengthen the immune system and reduce in ammation, potential y minimising psoriasis symptoms.

3. **Manage Stress:** Stress management techniques, such as mindfulness meditation, yoga, and deep breathing exercises, may help reduce stress levels and prevent psoriasis are-ups.

4. **Limit Alcohol and Smoking:** Alcohol consumption and smoking have been linked to an increased risk of psoriasis and may worsen existing symptoms. Limiting or avoiding these substances can help improve psoriasis management.

5. **Protect the Skin:** Use gentle skincare products, moisturise regularly, and avoid skin injuries, as trauma to the skin can trigger psoriasis are-ups.

Conclusion:

Psoriasis is a chronic autoimmune disorder that requires a multifaceted approach to diagnosis, prevention, and treatment. By accurately diagnosing the condition, identifying triggers, and implementing appropriate treatment strategies, healthcare providers can help patients e ectively manage their symptoms and improve their quality of life.

Through a combination of medical treatments, lifestyle modi cations, and ongoing support, individuals with psoriasis can achieve long-term symptom relief and minimise the impact of this chal enging condition.

Chapter-(4)

Lifestyle Management:

4.1:Diet and Nutrition.

4.2:Stress Management.

4.3:Skincare Tips.

4.4:Exercise and Physical Activity.

4.1:Diet and Nutrition.

With psoriasis, it's important to avoid foods that can trigger in ammation. In ammation and the immune system response can lead to a are-up.

When you have psoriasis, reducing triggers is an important part of managing your condition and avoiding are-ups. Psoriasis are-ups can be caused by a variety of triggers. These triggers may include bad weather, excess stress, and certain foods.

Let's take a look at the foods that are most likely to trigger a psoriasis are-up. There are some foods that are helpful to incorporate and certain diets to consider when creating a treatment plan for your psoriasis.

The foods listed below have been reported to trigger are-ups, but they may not a ect al those a ected by psoriasis.

Foods to avoid if you have psoriasis: Red meat and dairy

Red meat, dairy, and eggs contain a polyunsaturated fatty acid cal ed arachidonic acid. Past researchTrusted Source has shown that by-products of arachidonic acid may play a role in creating psoriatic lesions.

Foods to avoid include:

- red meat, especial y beef

- sausage, bacon, and other processed red meats

- eggs and egg

Gluten:

Celiac disease is a health condition characterised by an autoimmune response to the protein gluten. People with psoriasis have been found to have increased markers for gluten sensitivity. If you have psoriasis and a gluten sensitivity, it's important to cut out gluten-containing foods.

Foods to avoid include:

- wheat and wheat derivatives

- rye, barley, and malt

- pasta, noodles, and baked goods containing wheat, rye, barley, and malt

- certain processed foods

- certain sauces and condiments

- beer and malt beverages

Processed foods:

Eating too many processed, high-calorie foods can lead to obesity, metabolic syndrome, and a variety of chronic health conditions. Certain conditions such as these cause chronic in ammation in the body, which may be linkedTrusted Source to psoriasis are-ups.

Foods to avoid include:

- processed meats

- prepackaged food products

- canned fruits and vegetables

- any processed foods high in sugar, salt, and fat **Nightshades:**

One of the most commonly reported triggers for psoriasis are-ups is the consumption of nightshades.

Nightshade plants contain solanine, which has been known to a ect digestion and may be a cause of in ammationTrusted Source.

Foods to avoid include:

- tomatoes

- potatoes

- eggplants

- peppers

Alcohol:

Autoimmune are-ups are linked to the health of the immune system. Alcohol is believed to be a psoriasis trigger due to its disruptive e ects on the various pathways of the immune system. If you have psoriasis, it may be best to drink alcohol very sparingly.

Foods to eat if you have psoriasis: With psoriasis, a diet high in anti-in ammatory foods can help to reduce the severity of a are-up.

Fruits and vegetables:

Almost al anti-in ammatory diets include fruits and vegetables. Fruits and vegetables are high in antioxidants, which are compounds that decrease oxidative stress and in ammation. A diet high in fruits and vegetables is recommended for in ammatory conditions such as psoriasis.

Foods to eat include:

- broccoli, cauli ower, and Brussels sprouts

- leafy greens, such as kale, spinach, and arugula

- berries, including blueberries, strawberries, and raspberries

- cherries, grapes, and other dark fruits.

Fatty sh:

A diet high in fatty sh can provide the body with anti-in ammatory omega-3s. The intake of omega-3s has been linked to a decrease of in ammatory substances and overal in ammation.

Fish to eat include:

- salmon, fresh and canned

- sardines

- trout

- cod

It should be noted that there is stil more research that needs to be done on the link between omega-3s and psoriasis.

Heart-healthy oils:

Like fatty sh, certain oils also contain anti-in ammatory fatty acids. It's important to focus on oils that have a higher ratio of omega-3 to omega-6

fatty acids.

Oils to eat include:

- olive oil

- coconut oil

-

axseed oil

- sa ower oil.

Nutritional supplements:

A 2013 review of research literature showed that nutritional supplements may help reduce in ammation in psoriasis. Fish oil, vitamin D, vitamin B-12, and selenium have al been researched for psoriasis.

Bene ts of supplementation with these nutrients may include a decrease in the frequency and severity of are-ups.

4.2:Stress Management:

Stress and psoriasis often go hand in hand. Stress can make psoriasis worse, and psoriasis can make you feel stressed. But there are ways to ease stress that may help your psoriasis, too.

Understanding Psoriasis and Stress Stress, a common aspect of modern life, has been found to trigger or exacerbate psoriasis are-ups. The intricate relationship between stress and psoriasis is complex and multifaceted, involving both physiological and psychological factors.

Moreover, stress can also worsen the psychological impact of psoriasis. Dealing with the physical symptoms of psoriasis can take a tol on mental health, leading to feelings of anxiety, depression, and low self-esteem. The visible nature of psoriasis lesions can

also contribute to social stigma and isolation, further compounding the psychological burden.

The Link Between Psoriasis and Stress Research has shown that individuals with psoriasis experience higher levels of psychological stress compared to those without the condition. The chronic nature of psoriasis, the visible symptoms, and the unpredictability of are-ups can al contribute to heightened stress levels.

Furthermore, stress can create a vicious cycle with psoriasis. The stress caused by the condition itself can trigger are-ups, which in turn can lead to additional stress and worsen the symptoms. This cyclical relationship can make it chal enging for individuals with psoriasis to break free from the grip of stress.

It is important to note that stress does not cause psoriasis. Rather, it acts as a trigger or exacerbating factor for those who already have the condition.

Understanding this distinction is crucial in developing e ective management strategies.

How Stress Triggers Psoriasis Flare-Ups: The exact mechanisms through which stress triggers psoriasis are-ups are not ful y understood. However, researchers have identi ed several potential pathways that shed light on this intricate relationship.

One proposed mechanism involves stress hormones, such as cortisol, which play a role in the immune system dysfunction and in ammation that occur in psoriasis. Stress can disrupt the delicate balance of the immune system, leading to an overactive response that targets healthy skin cel s.

Additional y, stress can impair the body's natural healing processes and compromise the skin's barrier function. This makes the skin more susceptible to irritation and in ammation, further exacerbating psoriasis symptoms.

Furthermore, stress can in uence lifestyle factors that contribute to psoriasis are-ups. For instance, individuals under stress may engage in unhealthy coping mechanisms such as smoking, excessive alcohol consumption, or poor dietary choices. These behaviours can trigger or worsen psoriasis symptoms.

It is worth mentioning that stress management techniques, such as mindfulness meditation, exercise, and therapy, have been shown to help reduce psoriasis symptoms and improve overal wel -being. By addressing stress, individuals with psoriasis can potential y break the cycle and regain control over their condition.

Role of Stress Management in Preventing Psoriasis Flare-Ups:

By e ectively managing stress, individuals with psoriasis can reduce the triggers that may lead to are-ups. Stress management techniques can help modulate the body's in ammatory response and promote a healthier immune system.

Deep breathing:

One e ective stress management technique is deep breathing exercises. Deep breathing helps activate the body's relaxation response, reducing stress and promoting a sense of calm. By practising deep breathing regularly, individuals with psoriasis can lower their stress levels and potential y reduce the frequency of are-ups.

Physical activities:

Another helpful stress management technique is engaging in regular physical activity. Exercise has been shown to release endorphins, which are natural mood-boosting chemicals in the brain. Regular exercise can help reduce stress, improve overal wel -being, and potential y decrease the severity of psoriasis symptoms.

Mindfulness:

In addition to deep breathing exercises and regular physical activity, individuals with psoriasis can also bene t from practising mindfulness and meditation.

Mindfulness involves focusing on the present moment and accepting it without judgement. By practising

mindfulness, individuals with psoriasis can cultivate a sense of inner peace and reduce stress levels.

Support system:

Furthermore, seeking support from others can also be bene cial for managing stress in psoriasis care.

Connecting with support groups or talking to a therapist can provide individuals with psoriasis a safe space to express their emotions, share experiences, and learn coping strategies.

It is important to note that stress management techniques may vary for each individual. What works for one person may not work for another. It is essential for individuals with psoriasis to explore di erent stress management techniques and nd what works best for them

4.3:Skincare Tips for Psoriasis: Managing psoriasis requires a multifaceted approach, including skincare. Here are detailed skin care tips for psoriasis:

Moisturise Regularly: Keep your skin hydrated by applying moisturisers regularly, especial y after bathing or showering. Look for moisturisers that are fragrance-free and hypoal ergenic.

Use Gentle Cleansers: Opt for mild, fragrance-free cleansers that won't irritate your skin. Avoid harsh soaps and detergents, as they can worsen psoriasis symptoms.

Avoid Hot Water: Hot water can strip away natural oils from your skin, exacerbating psoriasis. Use lukewarm water for bathing and showering, and limit your time in the water.

Pat Dry, Don't Rub: After bathing or showering, gently pat your skin dry with a towel instead of rubbing it, which can irritate sensitive areas.

Avoid Scratching: Scratching can further in ame psoriasis plaques and lead to infection. Keep your nails short and consider wearing gloves at night to prevent scratching while you sleep.

Sun Protection:

While some sunlight can improve psoriasis symptoms, too much can trigger are-ups. Use sunscreen with a high SPF to protect your skin when outdoors, and consider wearing protective clothing and seeking shade.

Avoid Triggers: Identify and avoid triggers that worsen your psoriasis symptoms, such as stress, certain medications, alcohol, smoking, and certain foods.

Use Topical Treatments: Fol ow your doctor's recommendations for topical treatments, such as corticosteroids, coal tar, salicylic acid, or moisturisers containing ingredients like ceramides or urea.

Try Bathing Treatments:

Adding ingredients like col oidal oatmeal, Epsom salts, or Dead Sea salts to your bathwater can help soothe itchy, in amed skin.

However, avoid hot water and limit bathtime to prevent drying out your skin.

Manage Stress: Stress can trigger psoriasis are-ups, so incorporate stress-reducing techniques into your daily routine, such as mindfulness meditation, yoga, deep breathing exercises, or hobbies you enjoy.

Stay Hydrated:

Drink plenty of water to keep your skin hydrated from the inside out.

Consult Your Dermatologist:

Psoriasis is a chronic condition that may require medical management. Work closely with your dermatologist to develop a personalised skin care and treatment plan that meets your needs.

Remember, consistency is key when it comes to managing psoriasis. By incorporating these skincare

tips into your daily routine, you can help al eviate symptoms and improve the overal health of your skin.

4.4:Exercise and Physical Activity: Psoriasis is a chronic autoimmune condition characterised by in amed, red, scaly patches on the skin. While exercise and physical activity may not directly treat psoriasis, they can play a signi cant role in managing its symptoms and improving overal wel -being. Here's how:

Stress Reduction:

Exercise is known to reduce stress levels by releasing endorphins, the body's natural stress relievers. Stress is a common trigger for psoriasis are-ups, so managing stress through regular exercise can help minimise the frequency and severity of outbreaks.

Immune Function:

Regular physical activity can boost the immune system, potential y helping to regulate the immune responses that contribute to psoriasis. Exercise can also reduce in ammation throughout the body, which may help al eviate psoriasis symptoms.

Weight Management:

Obesity is a risk factor for psoriasis and can exacerbate symptoms. Exercise helps in weight management by burning calories and building muscle mass.

Maintaining a healthy weight through regular physical activity can reduce the severity of psoriasis symptoms and improve overal health.

Improved Circulation:

Exercise promotes better blood circulation, which is bene cial for people with psoriasis. Enhanced circulation can help deliver more oxygen and nutrients to the skin, promoting healing and reducing in ammation.

Mood Enhancement:

Living with a chronic condition like psoriasis can take a tol on mental health. Exercise has been shown to improve mood and reduce symptoms of depression and anxiety, which are common comorbidities of psoriasis.

Joint Health:

Psoriatic arthritis is a type of arthritis that a ects some people with psoriasis, causing joint pain and sti ness.

Exercise, particularly low-impact activities like swimming or yoga, can help maintain joint exibility and reduce pain associated with psoriatic arthritis.

Skin Health:

Sweating during exercise can help cleanse the skin and unclog pores, potential y reducing the risk of psoriasis are-ups. However, it's important to shower and

change into clean, dry clothes after exercising to prevent irritation or infection.

Quality of Life:

Engaging in regular physical activity can improve overal quality of life for people with psoriasis. It provides a sense of control over one's health, enhances self-esteem, and promotes social interaction if done in group settings.

It's essential for individuals with psoriasis to choose exercises that are suitable for their tness level and consider any limitations or sensitivities related to their condition. Consulting with a healthcare provider or a physical therapist can help develop a personalised exercise plan tailored to individual needs and goals.

Additional y, staying hydrated, wearing appropriate clothing, and protecting the skin from sun exposure are important considerations when incorporating exercise into a psoriasis management regimen.

Chapter-(5)

Alternative or Home Therapies:

5.1:Herbal Remedies

5.2:Acupuncture and Acupressure

5.3:Mind-Body Techniques.

5.1:Herbal Remedies:

Can herbal treatments help psoriasis symptoms?

Yes,Researchers are increasingly nding that herbal remedies real y can help relieve the symptoms of psoriasis.

But Herbal remedies for psoriasis should be used as a complement to the medications and treatments prescribed by your healthcare professional, not instead of the meds.

As per my own research ,there haven't been enough studies into herbal solutions yet. And until we know more, it's much better to use them for a little extra relief instead of your main treatment.

Science and nature go hand in hand. Make the most of both!

The six most e ective herbal treatments for psoriasis:

Let's check out these (possible) herbal heroes for psoriasis.

A. Oregon grape:

Oregon grapes (Berberis and Mahonia) have anti-in ammatory properties.

The stem and leaves of the plant can be ground into a powder or distil ed into an extract that is then used to make a topical skin cream. It's been found to reduce redness in psoriatic ares when used topical y.

In various clinical studies, skin creams containing 10%

Oregon grape extract were shown to be helpful in reducing psoriasis symptoms. The cream can cause itching and burning during the application in some cases.

The research is promising about Oregon grapes. A 2018 review looked at eight studies and found that Oregon grapes signi cantly improved psoriasis symptoms without causing side e ects.

It works by soothing in ammation of your skin and slowing down the growth of skin cel s, helping your patches simmer down and become less red.

Bear in mind that it's not a wonder cure and works best on psoriasis symptoms that are mild to moderate.

How to use;

You can buy Oregon grape as an oil, extract, tincture, capsule, or a cream and apply it directly to your skin.

B. Indigo naturalis:

This Chinese herb also goes under the name Qing-Dai.

Indigo is a traditional medicine that actual y has some science on its side.

Qing Dai (Indigo) is a plant used in traditional Chinese medicine. It's also been used to make indigo-coloured dye for many centuries.

In various older clinical studies, creams containing 10%

Indigo naturalist extract reduced psoriasis symptoms by 81%in some cases compared with placebo treatment, though this depended on the dose and speci c composition.

A newer 2017 study found that 56.3% of participants had a 75% improvement in treatment.

How to use:

Indigo is available in creams for topical use. It also comes in handy bottles that al ow you to dab it onto your nails if psoriasis has shown itself there.

C.Aloe vera (Aloe vera barbadensis):

Aloe vera is a plant known for its soothing and cooling properties. Aloe vera may also help regenerate skin cel s and heal irritated skin.

It has also been shown to help reduce symptoms of mild-to-moderate psoriasis through various studies.

Truth is that there's less evidence available to show that aloe vera can help people manage their psoriasis than either Oregon grape or Indigo . But that's not to say it won't do anything.

A 2019 review of studies suggests that some folks with psoriasis nd relief after using aloe vera, but it's less likely to have a signi cant e ect. Aloe does provide a nice cooling sensation and antibacterial properties, which is always useful — but it might not have a

super noteworthy impact on your symptoms.

D.Turmeric:

Turmeric (Curcuma longa) is part of the same family as the ginger plant. Its active ingredient is curcumin, and it has unique anti-in ammatory and antibacterial properties that have led scientists to study it as a treatment for psoriasis.

Recent studies are showing promise, with curcumin possibly being able to reduce your body's in ammatory response.Through various mechanisms of action, it has been shown to help with reducing psoriasis symptoms.

How to use;

you'l nd a fair few creams at your local drugstore and online that have turmeric as their main ingredient.

Closely fol ow the instructions when applying it to your skin.

There are also some turmeric essential oils that have a much higher concentration than the creams. But be sure to dilute them in a carrier oil rst.

E.Capsaicin:

Capsaicin is the active ingredient in chil i peppers (Capsicum). It's the reason you feel a burning sensation when you eat food seasoned with chilies.

The ability to create a "burning" of cel s might actual y help heal psoriasis ares, as wel as reduce the feeling of pain or itch.

F.Female ginseng:

Dong Quai (Angelica sinensis) is another herb used as a remedy in Chinese medicine.

It contains psoralen, which is the same compound you would consume before undergoing phototherapy.

Eating it before exposure to UV light can help reduce psoriasis symptoms.

There's also some evidence that just applying it topical y can help reduce skin itching related to atopic

dermatitis, which may mean it could o er some relief with other skin disorders like psoriasis.

you should never apply herbs and expose yourself to the sun without medical supervision or without consulting with a dermatologist rst. It's safer to use under Medical supervision through light therapy.

G.Apple Cider Vinegar for Your Scalp: Apple Cider Vinegar is more than just a salad dressing.

Put some on your head a few times a week -- either ful strength or mixed with water. It's a recipe for relief when your scalp cal s out "scratch me."

Rinse it o after it dries so you won't get an irritation.

And don't try this when your scalp is bleeding or cracked. The vinegar wil make it feel like it's burning.

H.Other herbs:

suggests that other herbs might have properties that may be helpful for psoriasis.

They include:

- fennel (Foeniculum vulgare)

- anise (Pimpinel a)

- clove (Syzygium aromaticum)

- basil (Ocimum basilicum)

- araroba tree (Stereopsis araroba)

- barberry bark (Mahonia)

- gotu kola (Centel a asiatica L.)

- day blooming jasmine (Cestrum diurnum)

- American wintergreen (Gaultheria

procumbens L.)

- Khel a (Ammi visnaga L.)

- Queen Anne's lace (Ammi majus L.)

- German chamomile (Matricaria L.)

- narrow-leaved paperbark (Melaleuca)

- black seed (Nigel a sativa)

- olibanum (Boswel ia serrata)

5.2:Acupuncture and Acupressure: A)Acupuncture Treatment:

Acupuncture is a type of alternative medicine that originated in ancient China. It involves the insertion of thin needles into speci c points on the body to promote healing and al eviate pain. According to traditional Chinese medicine, acupuncture works by balancing the ow of energy, also known as Qi, throughout the body.

According to scientists and researchers, the e ectiveness of acupuncture treatment lies in its ability to stimulate the body's natural healing mechanisms.

The insertion of thin needles into speci c points on the skin triggers the release of neurotransmitters and hormones that regulate pain, emotions, and immunity.

Additional y, acupuncture may also improve blood ow, reduce in ammation, and activate neural pathways that al eviate symptoms. While some clinical trials have shown promising results, the scienti c evidence for acupuncture's e cacy is stil inconclusive, and more research is needed to establish its safety and long-term bene ts.

Nevertheless, many people have reported positive outcomes from acupuncture, and it continues to be a viable treatment option for those seeking alternative therapies.

Is Acupuncture for Psoriasis Bene cial?

Acupuncture for psoriasis works by stimulating the body's natural healing processes and promoting balance in the immune system. The needles are inserted into speci c points on the body that correspond to di erent organs and systems, such as the liver, spleen, and kidneys. By targeting these points, acupuncture can help reduce in ammation, improve circulation,

and boost the immune system, al of which can help al eviate psoriasis symptoms. Acupuncture can also help reduce stress and anxiety, which are common triggers for psoriasis are-ups.

What are the Bene ts of Acupuncture for Psoriasis?

Acupuncture has been shown to have numerous bene ts for those with psoriasis. It can help reduce in ammation, improve circulation, and boost the immune system, al of which can help al eviate psoriasis symptoms. Acupuncture also has positive e ects on mental wel -being, which is essential for psoriasis su erers. Acupuncture is a natural and holistic approach to healing that can be used in conjunction with other treatments for psoriasis. It is a safe and e ective way to manage symptoms and improve overal health and wel -being.

Are there any Side e ects to Acupuncture for Psoriasis?

Acupuncture is general y considered safe when performed by a licensed practitioner. However, some people may experience mild side e ects such as: **1. Bruising and soreness at the insertion site**: The insertion of needles into the skin can cause bruising

and soreness, which may last for a few days fol owing treatment.

2. Fatigue: Some people may experience feelings of fatigue or tiredness fol owing acupuncture treatment.

This is thought to be due to changes in hormone levels and increased blood ow.

3. Dizziness or lightheadedness: In rare cases, people may experience dizziness or lightheadedness during or fol owing acupuncture treatment. This is usual y temporary and can be resolved by lying down or resting.

4. Infection: There is a smal risk of infection at the insertion site if proper hygiene and sterilisation procedures are not fol owed. However, this risk is very low when acupuncture is performed by a licensed and experienced practitioner.

Reviews Suggesting Acupuncture Therapies For Psoriasis Treatment:

In a systematic review conducted in 2015, the authors found trace evidence of acupuncture being bene cial for managing psoriasis symptoms. However, they also admitted that the review was based on a smal amount of randomised control ed trials and few cases had con icting results.

Another overview of literature in 2016 claims that undertaking acupuncture treatment of psoriasis could be e ective involving minimal side e ects.

Yet another review conducted in 2017 involved the use of a randomised control ed trial done 13 times only to state that acupuncture-related techniques like acupressure can be accepted as a complementary and alternative therapy for psoriasis, encouraging further research.

B)How acupressure treats psoriasis: Acupressure is a traditional Chinese medicine technique that involves applying pressure to speci c points on the body to al eviate symptoms and promote healing. While acupressure can provide relief for some symptoms associated with psoriasis, such as itching and in ammation, it's important to note that it's not a cure for the condition itself.

Here's how acupressure may help with psoriasis: **Stress Reduction**: Stress is known to exacerbate psoriasis symptoms. Acupressure targets speci c pressure points to promote relaxation and reduce stress levels, which may help al eviate symptoms associated with psoriasis.

Improving Blood Circulation: Acupressure stimulates blood circulation throughout the body. By improving blood ow to the skin, it may help reduce in ammation and promote healing of psoriatic lesions.

Balancing Qi: According to traditional Chinese medicine, psoriasis is believed to be caused by an imbalance of Qi, or life energy, in the body.

Acupressure aims to restore the balance of Qi by applying pressure to speci c points along energy channels known as meridians.

Boosting Immune Function: Some proponents of acupressure believe that stimulating certain pressure points can enhance the body's immune function, which may help al eviate symptoms of autoimmune conditions like psoriasis.

It's essential to consult with a quali ed acupuncturist or healthcare professional before attempting acupressure, especial y if you have underlying health conditions or are pregnant. While acupressure can complement conventional treatments for psoriasis, it should not replace medical advice or prescribed treatments.

5.3:Mind-Body Techniques to treat psoriasis: Mind-body techniques can complement traditional medical treatments for psoriasis by addressing the

psychological and emotional aspects of the condition.

Some of these techniques include:

Stress Management: Stress is a known trigger for psoriasis are-ups. Mind-body techniques such as deep breathing exercises, progressive muscle relaxation, and mindfulness meditation can help reduce stress levels, thereby potential y decreasing the frequency and severity of psoriasis symptoms.

Cognitive Behavioral Therapy (CBT): CBT is a type of psychotherapy that helps individuals identify and change negative thought patterns and behaviours.

It can be bene cial for people with psoriasis by addressing feelings of embarrassment, shame, or low self-esteem associated with the condition.

Biofeedback: Biofeedback is a technique that teaches individuals to control involuntary bodily processes such as heart rate, muscle tension, and skin temperature. By learning to regulate these physiological responses, people with psoriasis may be able to reduce stress and improve their overal wel -being.

Hypnotherapy: Hypnotherapy involves inducing a state of deep relaxation and heightened suggestibility to promote positive changes in behaviour or perception.

While more research is needed, some studies suggest that hypnotherapy may help al eviate psoriasis symptoms by reducing stress and enhancing immune function.

Visualisation and Guided Imagery: Visualization and guided imagery techniques involve mental y

visualising peaceful and calming scenes to promote relaxation and reduce stress. This can help people with psoriasis manage their symptoms and cope with the emotional impact of the condition.

Yoga and Tai Chi: Yoga and Tai Chi are mind-body practices that combine physical postures, breathing exercises, and meditation. These practices can improve exibility, strength, and balance while also promoting relaxation and stress reduction, which may bene t individuals with psoriasis.

It's important to note that while mind-body techniques can be helpful for managing psoriasis symptoms, they should not replace medical treatment prescribed by a healthcare professional. It's essential to work with a quali ed therapist or practitioner to determine which techniques are most appropriate for your individual needs and circumstances.

Chapter-(6)

Research and Future Directions:

6.1:Latest Developments in Psoriasis Research.

6.2:Promising Treatments on the Horizon.

6.1:Latest Developments in Psoriasis Research: As more than eight mil ion people in the U.S. alone live with psoriasis, there is a need for broader treatment approaches. Typical y, patients with psoriasis, who experience symptoms like skin lesions, which may be sore and itchy, are prescribed topical creams, phototherapy – where light is used to slow down the production of skin cel s – and biological medicines that target in ammation. Since many of the creams are steroid-based – where side e ects like early onset skin thinning accompany their e ectiveness – biotech companies are in pursuit of anti-in ammatory therapies that have fewer side e ects.

As we observe Psoriasis Awareness Month in August, let us take a look at ve recent advancements in psoriasis research over the past year.

a)New class of drug to treat plaque psoriasis gains approval:

The rst-ever al osteric tyrosine kinase 2 (TYK2) inhibitor was approved by the U.S. Food and Drug Administration (FDA) for the treatment of plaque psoriasis, which a ects nearly 90% of patients diagnosed with psoriasis, last September. The drug, , sold under the brand name *Sotyktu*, by American multinational pharmaceutical company Bristol Myers Squibb, was given the go ahead after the drug was successful in phase 3 clinical trials.

The trials, POETYK PSO-1 and POETYK PSO-2, found the once-daily oral to be e cacious in 1,684

patients against a placebo. The e ectiveness of the drug was observed 16 and 24 weeks after dosage, and persisted through 52 weeks. Moreover, patients had a comparatively greater positive response than when treated with American multinational biopharma Amgen's Otezla.

"The approval of Sotyktu represents an exciting day for patients su ering from moderate-to-severe plaque psoriasis who are not satis ed with topical and conventional treatments. Sotyktu works by inhibiting an enzyme and disrupting a cytokine pathway that triggers in ammation. While the drug proved to have improved symptoms of psoriasis, during clinical trials, 2.4% of patients discontinued the drug because of serious adverse reactions, compared to 3.8% in the

placebo group, and more than 5% who were given Otezla.

b)Research nds a new drug delivery strategy could target psoriasis better:

The S100A9 gene's link to psoriasis has long been at the centre of autoimmune disease research. Now, research conducted by the Medical University of Vienna has worked out that the severity of psoriasis can be relieved by inhibiting the expression of the gene throughout the whole body, instead of just on the skin.

The study, which took place last year, led by biochemist Erwin Wagner, from the Department of Dermatology and Department of Laboratory Medicine at MedUni Vienna, aimed to investigate the signi cance of S100A9, in causing psoriasis symptoms.

"Our study is an important step towards the development of targeted therapeutic options in the form of drugs that act systemical y rather than local y on the skin," said Wagner.

This comes after Wagner's team found that when the gene was inactivated in al the cel s in the body, symptoms experienced by patients with psoriasis had reduced. This research could enable pharmaceuticals to reconsider and adapt drug delivery accordingly – this

could be in the form of tablets or drops – to obtain the best therapeutic results.

c)Boehringer Ingelheim receives FDA nod for psoriasis drug:

A rare form of psoriasis, generalised pustular psoriasis (GPP), as the name suggests, leads to pus- l ed blisters on the body. These are ups are often triggered by stress, infections, exposure to too much ultraviolet (UV) light and certain medication like steroids.

Typical y, treatments include anti-in ammatory drugs as wel as biologics such as adalimumab. With the FDA's clearance of , almost a year ago, treatment approaches have widened.

Sold under the name Spevigo, German pharmaceutical Boehringer Ingelheim's drug is a monoclonal antibody that binds to and blocks IL-36, a protein receptor that prompts in ammation when overexpressed. The approval came fol owing a promising trial, where out of 53 patients, 54% of them were free of the pus- l ed bumps after one week of having received a single dose of the drug, compared to 6% in the placebo group.

"GPP ares may appear suddenly, intensify quickly, and can be life-threatening if left untreated, leaving those a ected feeling anxious and uncertain about their future," said Carinne Brouil on, member of the Board of Managing Directors and head of Human Pharma at

Boehringer Ingelheim. "The FDA's recognition of the urgent need for preventing GPP ares is a major step towards empowering people living with the condition to plan critical moments in their lives, despite their disease."

Later, in December last year, the drug was authorised for conditional marketing by the European Commission, granting its sale across the European Union (EU).

d)Research unveils link between dietary fats and psoriasis symptoms:

Linoleic acid, a type of fatty acid present in nuts, seeds and vegetable oils, is a big part of the Western diet. A study carried out by North Carolina State University in the U.S., was able to derive a link between the fatty acid and lesions caused by psoriasis.

"We noticed high levels of two types of lipids derived from linoleic acid in psoriatic lesions," said Santosh Mishra, author of the study and associate professor of neuroscience at North Carolina State University.

This discovery led the team to wonder whether these lipids impacted the way the neurons in the lesions communicated. Using mass spectrometry, they created lipid pro les of the skin's psoriatic ares. Linoleic acid-derived lipids in particular, were found to have not only bound to the sensory neuron receptors present in the skin, but also had a prolonged e ect compared to oxy lipids – another kind of lipid that was examined.

Once bound to the receptors, the lipids activate two sets of neuronal receptors, namely TRPA1 and TRPV1. These receptors play a major role in control ing hypersensitivity to temperature and pain, major symptoms experienced by people with psoriasis.

"We know that this lipid moves from one form to another, but don't yet know what causes that,"

commented Mishra. "We also know what protein the lipids are binding to, but not where the bond occurs.

Answering these questions may hopeful y lead to new therapies – or dietary solutions – for some psoriasis su erers."

This recent nding could drive further research to relieve these symptoms for those a ected by psoriasis.

e)Non-steroidal topical cream with limited side e ects wins FDA approval:

An anti-in ammatory medicine, *roflumilast* is used to treat people with chronic obstructive pulmonary disease (COPD). Now, it is being prescribed in the U.S.

for plaque psoriasis, after the FDA gave the green light last year.

California-based Arcutis Biotherapeutics' ro umilast cream (ZORREVE) joins to expand non-steroidal topical medication options, but is regarded as a one-of-a-kind treatment as it is the rst PDE4 inhibitor to be approved. PDE-4 inhibitors work by curbing the production of the enzyme PDE-4, which sometimes gets in the way of certain chemical reactions, setting o in ammation. To this, the skin responds adversely, by hyping up skin cel growth of plaque psoriasis.

The approval was led by encouraging results from two phase 3 clinical trials published in the Journal of the American Medical Association. The cream was found to be e ective in intertriginous areas – regions of skin folds, where the skin rubs against each other – and, based on the psoriasis area severity index (PASI), 40%

of the patients achieved a 75% reduction in PASI scores by the eighth week. Moreover, patients who experienced severe itching, had a four-point decline on the worst itch numerical rating scale (WI-NRS). Also, the treatment did not cause drastic side e ects and was found to be tolerable.

"Coupled with ZORYVE's favourable safety and tolerability data, these results reinforce that ZORYVE

can o er patients a single topical therapy for use on al psoriasis-a ected areas – including hard to treat areas such as elbows and knees and intertriginous areas.

6.2:Promising Treatments on the Horizon: Psoriasis is mediated by pro-in ammatory cytokine.One of the main cytokines that plays a role in this and other autoimmune diseases is IL-17.

The landscape of psoriasis treatments has undergone rapid change within the last decade and the dizzying speed of drug development has not slowed, with 4

notable entries into the psoriasis treatment armamentarium within the last year: , ro umilast, , and

. Several others are in late-stage development, and these therapies represent new mechanisms, pathways, and delivery systems, meaningful y broadening the spectrum of treatment choices for our patients.

However, it can be quite di cult to keep track of al the medication options. This review aims to present the mechanisms and data on both newly available therapeutics for psoriasis and products in the pipeline that may have a notable impact on our treatment paradigm for psoriasis in the near future.

Here is the overview of some promising treatments for psoriasis.

● *Roflumilast, a phosphodiesterase 4 inhibitor, and an aryl hydrocarbon receptor–modulating agent, are 2 novel nonsteroidal topical treatments safe for regular long-term use on all affected areas of the skin in adult patients with plaque psoriasis.*

● *Deucravacitinib*

is an oral selective tyrosine kinase 2 allosteric inhibitor that has demonstrated a favourable safety profile and greater levels of efficacy than other available oral medications for plaque psoriasis.

● *The dual inhibition of IL-17A and IL-17F*

provides faster responses and greater clinical benefits for patients with moderate to severe plaque psoriasis than inhibition of IL-17A alone, achieving higher levels of efficacy than has been reported with any other biologic therapy.

● *Spesolimab, an IL-36 receptor inhibitor, is an effective, US Food and Drug*

Administration–approved treatment for patients with generalised pustular psoriasis.

While there's stil no cure for psoriasis, new science and medications are making great headway in better control ing the condition, giving our psoriasis patients renewed hope.

Here, we review three of these promising therapies and how they can help you reclaim your life when you have psoriasis.

1. Biologics;

Until recently, our best defence against psoriasis was in treating the symptoms (more on this in a moment).

While e ective, these treatments didn't address the

underlying autoimmune disorder, which is not only responsible for the in ammation and plaques in your skin, but it can lead to psoriatic arthritis and cardiovascular issues, as wel .

For a more systemic approach to psoriasis, we're now leaning on biologics, which go straight to the heart of the problem — your immune system. Made from human or animal proteins, these medications quiet your hyperactive immune cel s by blocking the most potent pro-in ammatory biochemical interleukin-17

— IL-17A.

The FDA has approved several of these biologics, including secukinumab (Cosentyx®) and adalimumab (Humira®), but a new biologic is poised to be even more e ective — .

This biologic targets your IL-17A like the others, but goes a step further as it also addresses your IL-17F, which isn't as powerful as IL-17A, but this chemical is plentiful.

Early clinical trials have shown to be very successful.

One trial was conducted at 77 sites around the world and involved people with moderate to severe psoriasis.

After receiving either a placebo, the patients who received experienced a 90% reduction in plaques in

four months. And with further maintenance dosing, these patients maintained their results over 56 weeks **2. Light therapy;**

We've also had great success in reducing the in ammatory responses in the skin with light therapy.

With this innovative technology, we deliver ultraviolet B rays into your skin, which target and slow the cel s that create the visible signs of psoriasis.

3. Retinoids;

Another great way to manage the plaques and rashes on your skin is through retinoid therapy. Retinoids are synthetic forms of vitamin A that can slow the growth of rapidly growing skin cel s, lessen redness, and reduce thick plaques of psoriasis.

While you can buy over-the-counter retinols, they aren't general y e ective for psoriasis.

Chapter-(7)

Conclusion:

7.1:Staying Positive and Hopeful.

7.2:Moving Forward in Your Journey.

7.1:Staying Positive and Hopeful.

Living with psoriasis can be chal enging, but there are strategies to help you stay positive and hopeful: 1. **Educate Yourself:** Understanding your condition can empower you to manage it better. Learn about psoriasis, its triggers, treatments, and lifestyle changes that can help.

2. **Focus on What You Can Control:** While you can't control having psoriasis, you can control how you manage it. Focus on healthy habits like maintaining a balanced diet, exercising regularly, and managing stress.

3. **Connect with Others:** Join support groups or online communities where you can connect with others who understand what you're going through. Sharing experiences and advice can be uplifting.

4. **Practice Self-Care:** Make time for activities that help you relax and feel good about yourself, whether it's taking a warm bath,

practising mindfulness, or pursuing a hobby you enjoy.

5. **Set Realistic Goals:** Break down large goals into smal er, achievable steps. Celebrate your progress along the way, no matter how smal .

6. **Seek Professional Help**: Don't hesitate to reach out to healthcare professionals for support. They can provide guidance on managing your condition and o er treatment options tailored to your needs.

7. **Stay Optimistic:** Remember that psoriasis doesn't de ne you. Focus on your strengths, accomplishments, and the things that bring you joy in life.

8. **Stay Persistent**: Managing psoriasis is often a journey with ups and downs. Stay committed to your treatment plan and lifestyle changes, and don't get discouraged by setbacks.

By adopting these strategies, you can cultivate a positive outlook and maintain hope while living with psoriasis.

7.2:Moving Forward in Your Journey.

Moving forward in your journey with psoriasis involves several key steps:

Educate Yourself: Learn as much as you can about psoriasis, its causes, symptoms, and available

treatments. Understanding your condition wil empower you to make informed decisions about managing it.

Consult a Healthcare Professional: Work closely with a dermatologist or healthcare provider specialising in psoriasis. They can provide personalised treatment plans and monitor your progress over time.

Develop a Treatment Plan: Discuss various treatment options with your healthcare provider, including topical treatments, phototherapy, oral medications, and biologic therapies. Together, you can create a plan that addresses your speci c needs and goals.

Establish a Skincare Routine: Develop a daily skincare routine to help manage psoriasis symptoms and prevent are-ups. This may include gentle cleansing, moisturising, and using prescribed medications as directed.

Maintain a Healthy Lifestyle: Aim to adopt healthy habits such as eating a balanced diet, exercising regularly, managing stress, and getting enough sleep.

These lifestyle factors can play a signi cant role in managing psoriasis and promoting overal wel -being.

Monitor and Manage Triggers: Pay attention to factors that may trigger or exacerbate your psoriasis symptoms, such as stress, certain foods, weather changes, or medications. Take steps to minimise exposure to these triggers whenever possible.

Seek Support: Connect with others who have psoriasis through support groups, online forums, or social media communities. Sharing experiences and tips with others can provide valuable support and encouragement along your journey.

Stay Positive and Patient:

Managing psoriasis is often a lifelong journey with ups and downs. Stay positive and patient, and remember that with proper management and support, you can lead a ful l ing life despite psoriasis.